Occupation-Based
Activity Analysis
SECOND EDITION

Occupation-Based
Activity Analysis
SECOND EDITION

Heather Thomas, PhD, OTR/L

Associate Professor and Curriculum Coordinator
West Coast University
Los Angeles, California

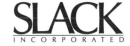

www.Healio.com/books

ISBN: 978-1-61711-967-5

Occupation-Based Activity Analysis, Second Edition includes ancillary materials specifically available for faculty use. Included are PowerPoint slides and handouts. Please visit www.efacultylounge.com to obtain access.

Dr. Heather Thomas has no financial or proprietary interest in the materials presented herein.

The procedures and practices described in this publication should be implemented in a manner consistent with the professional standards set for the circumstances that apply in each specific situation. Every effort has been made to confirm the accuracy of the information presented and to correctly relate generally accepted practices. The authors, editors, and publisher cannot accept responsibility for errors or exclusions or for the outcome of the material presented herein. There is no expressed or implied warranty of this book or information imparted by it. Care has been taken to ensure that drug selection and dosages are in accordance with currently accepted/recommended practice. Off-label uses of drugs may be discussed. Due to continuing research, changes in government policy and regulations, and various effects of drug reactions and interactions, it is recommended that the reader carefully review all materials and literature provided for each drug, especially those that are new or not frequently used. Some drugs or devices in this publication have clearance for use in a restricted research setting by the Food and Drug and Administration or FDA. Each professional should determine the FDA status of any drug or device prior to use in their practice.

Any review or mention of specific companies or products is not intended as an endorsement by the author or publisher.

SLACK Incorporated uses a review process to evaluate submitted material. Prior to publication, educators or clinicians provide important feedback on the content that we publish. We welcome feedback on this work.

Published by: SLACK Incorporated
                    6900 Grove Road
                    Thorofare, NJ 08086 USA
                    Telephone: 856-848-1000
                    Fax: 856-848-6091
                    www.Healio.com/books

Contact SLACK Incorporated for more information about other books in this field or about the availability of our books from distributors outside the United States.

Library of Congress Cataloging-in-Publication Data

Thomas, Heather, 1971- , author.
  Occupation-based activity analysis / Heather Thomas. -- Second edition.
     p. ; cm.
  Includes bibliographical references and index.
  ISBN 978-1-61711-967-5 (paperback)
  I. Title.
  [DNLM: 1. Occupational Therapy--methods. 2. Activities of Daily Living. 3. Psychomotor Performance. 4. Treatment Outcome. WB 555]
  RM735
  615.8'515--dc23
                    2015014977

Printed in the United States of America.

Last digit is print number: 10 9 8

Dedication

So much of what we become is based on what we know is possible. My parents knew no limits to my future and encouraged me through all of the adventures I have taken on, including the writing of this book. Thank you for continually encouraging me and providing the occasional reminder to slow down. Your guidance has brought me to where I am today.

To all of my friends, my patient husband, and past students, thank you for allowing me to "disappear" for hours (and days) at a time to write. Some of you were kind enough to allow me to follow you around with a camera, which I greatly appreciate. I know you were thinking, "She wants a picture of me doing that?"

Finally, this book is dedicated to and written with great thanks to all occupational therapy students around the globe. The future of our profession lies in your hands, and the future is bright.

Contents

Acknowledgments

It is through engagement in occupations, and watching others engage in occupations, that I have come to truly understand the complexities of what we do every day. I would like to thank those who have given me a window into their occupations and daily lives—a brief insight into how and why activities occur. For this opportunity, I especially thank the clients I have served over the years. Your patience and trust have allowed me to learn about occupations beyond my own.

Heather Thomas, PhD, OTR/L

About the Author

Heather Thomas, PhD, OTR/L is an associate professor at West Coast University in Los Angeles, California. She began teaching activity analysis in 2004 at Loma Linda University. After obtaining her master's degree in occupational therapy from the University of Southern California in 1998, she studied health care administration at Touro University International in Cypress, California, and gained her PhD in health science in 2011. Thomas's clinical work focuses on the adult acute and acute rehabilitation settings. From 2000 to 2002, she was director of the Casa Colina Assistive Technology Center, and from 2007 to 2008, she served as director of Occupational Therapy Services at Casa Colina Centers for Rehabilitation in Pomona, California. She has served in multiple leadership roles within the Occupational Therapy Association of California and has presented at conferences of the American Occupational Therapy Association (AOTA). She currently serves as the California representative on the AOTA Representative Assembly. She has also served several terms as the chair of the Los Angeles Occupational Therapy Leadership Forum. Expanding occupational therapy's reach into underserved areas, she has volunteered in Haiti to work with those who were injured during the earthquake of 2010 and then helped develop a rehabilitation technician program in that country. A yoga instructor for many years, she now enjoys practicing yoga at home in Los Angeles, snow skiing, gardening, teaching, and learning new occupations.

Introduction

As a profession that uses occupations and activities as not only our goal, but also as a treatment medium, we must understand both the uniqueness of a client's occupations and how an activity can be used therapeutically. This text is an introduction to both realms, first by explaining the process by which to peel back the layers to reveal the intricacy of an activity and then examining how to use this information for evaluation and intervention. It is through this deep analysis that we come to understand how rich occupations can be.

It is through the process of writing this book that I have come to truly appreciate the vast difference between activities and occupations. To analyze the complexity of an occupation takes so much more depth of understanding of the person engaging in it, his or her environment, and the uniqueness of the occupation that the person has chosen. (How truly the "person, environment, occupation" model fits as a way of understanding occupation-based activity analysis!) As in an activity analysis, occupation-based analysis looks at what is required for full participation, yet it goes beyond analyzing the activity; it looks at what it means for the person engaging in it and how and where it is performed by that person.

The format for activity analysis in this text follows the activity demands section of the *Occupational Therapy Practice Framework, 3rd Edition* (or *Framework*; AOTA, 2014). The terminology used by the creators of this document comes from the International Classification of Functioning, Disability, and Health published by the World Health Organization (2001), as well as previously published occupational therapy literature. The term *demands* sets forth the idea that activities require something from those who participate and from elements within the environment for the activity to occur. It is interesting that the word *demands* was chosen and not *needed* or *requested*, which are much more passive terms.

This text addressed the following educational standards set by the Accreditation Council for Occupational Therapy Education (ACOTE) for doctoral and master's level and occupational therapy assistant programs:

- B.2.2 Explain (or describe) the meaning and dynamics of occupation and activity, including the interaction of areas of occupation, performance skills, performance patterns, activity demands, context(s) and environments, and client factors. (ACOTE, 2014, p. 19)

- B.2.3 Articulate to consumers, potential employers, colleagues, third-party payers, regulatory boards, policymakers, other audiences, and the general public both the unique nature of occupation as viewed by the profession of occupational therapy and the value of occupation to support performance, participation, health, and well-being. (ACOTE, 2014, p. 19)

- B.2.7 Demonstrate task analysis in areas of occupation, performance skills, performance patterns, activity demands, context(s) and environments, and client factors to formulate an intervention plan. (ACOTE, 2014, p. 20)

- B.4.10 Document occupational therapy services to ensure accountability of service provision and to meet standards for reimbursement of services, adhering to the requirements of applicable facility, local, state, federal, and reimbursement agencies. Documentation must effectively communicate the need and rationale for occupational therapy services. (ACOTE, 2014, p. 22)

- B.5.1 For Master's Degree: Use evaluation findings based on appropriate theoretical approaches, models of practice, and frames of reference to develop occupation-based intervention plans and strategies (including goals and methods to achieve them) on the basis of the stated needs of the client as well as data gathered during the evaluation process in collaboration with the client and others. Intervention plans and strategies must be culturally relevant, reflective of current occupational therapy practice, and based on available evidence. Interventions address the following components:
  - The occupational profile, including participation in activities that are meaningful and necessary for the client to carry out roles in home, work, and community environments.

- ○ Client factors, including values, beliefs, spirituality, body functions (e.g., neuromuscular, sensory and pain, visual, perceptual, cognitive, mental), and body structures (e.g., cardiovascular, digestive, nervous, genitourinary, integumentary systems).
  - ○ Performance patterns (e.g., habits, routines, rituals, roles). Context (e.g., cultural, personal, temporal, virtual) and environment (e.g., physical, social).
  - ○ Performance skills, including motor and praxis skills, sensory–perceptual skills, emotional regulation skills, cognitive skills, and communication and social skills. (ACOTE, 2014, p. 23-24)
- B.5.1 For Associate Degrees: Assist with the development of occupation-based intervention plans and strategies (including goals and methods to achieve them) on the basis of the stated needs of the client as well as data gathered during the evaluation process in collaboration with the client and others. Intervention plans and strategies must be culturally relevant, reflective of current occupational therapy practice, and based on available evidence. Interventions address the following components:
  - ○ The occupational profile, including participation in activities that are meaningful and necessary for the client to carry out roles in home, work, and community environments.
  - ○ Client factors, including values, beliefs, spirituality, body functions (e.g., neuromuscular, sensory and pain, visual, perceptual, cognitive, mental) and body structures (e.g., cardiovascular, digestive, nervous, genitourinary, integumentary systems).
  - ○ Performance patterns (e.g., habits, routines, rituals, roles).
  - ○ Context (e.g., cultural, personal, temporal, virtual) and environment (e.g., physical, social).
  - ○ Performance skills, including motor and praxis skills, sensory–perceptual skills, emotional regulation skills, cognitive skills, and communication and social skills. (ACOTE, 2014, p. 23-24)
- B.5.2 Select and provide direct occupational therapy interventions and procedures to enhance safety, health and wellness, and performance in ADLs, IADLs, education, work, play, rest, sleep, leisure, and social participation. (ACOTE, 2014, p. 24)
- B.5.9 Adapt environments (e.g., home, work, school, community) and processes, including the application of ergonomic principles. (ACOTE, 2014, p. 24)
- B.5.23 Grade and adapt the environment, tools, materials, occupations, and interventions to reflect the changing needs of the client, the sociocultural context, and technological advances. (ACOTE, 2014, p. 26)

As a foundational skill, activity analysis is utilized throughout students' careers and into their lives as practitioners. Over the years of teaching activity analysis, I have seen students refer back to their notes from activity analysis class to formulate answers to questions and problems posed in other classes. Students were using these notes, which defined areas of the *Framework*, as a reference. So it is the hope that this text will serve as a reference for future work in occupational therapy curricula, as it details the *Framework* and essential foundational information.

As an activity analysis text, this book should be read in the order in which the chapters appear. Starting with Chapter 1, the reader is led through the steps of analyzing an activity. The layout of the chapters reflects the process whereby activity analysis is typically completed. If one were to skip ahead to further chapters, the process might not be as clear and aspects of the activity might not be determined.

For use as a reference text, each chapter is designed to cover a particular aspect of the *Framework*. The areas of occupation listed in Table 1 of the *Framework* are described in Chapter 2. The body functions, part of the client factors that are part of Table 2 in the *Framework*, are explained in detail in Chapter 6. Body structures are also considered among the client factors and are described in Chapter 7. Chapters 3 and 4 cover much of the activity demands section of the *Framework*, located in Table 7. A review of the performance skills from Table 3 of the *Framework* is presented in Chapter 8 of the text.

To truly understand how to analyze activities, it is important to participate in the exercises and activities presented throughout the chapters. The ability to conduct analyses comes with practice, putting the knowledge gained to work. While information presented in this text provides a foundation, readers will gain a broader understanding of body functions and skills as their education and experience continue.

As you read this book, I hope that you will begin to look at the world through a new lens and begin to see how a "simple" activity may not be so simple—that every task has multiple factors that lead to successful participation. Our world is full of occupations that range in complexity and demand an insurmountable combination of body functions and skills. It is up to us as occupational therapy practitioners to be able to fully understand how the demands of those occupations fit with our clients and their contexts. Through this, we gain an understanding of how participation can be improved or enhanced.

Revisions made to the present volume:

After the third edition of the *Occupational Therapy Practice Framework* was released in April 2014, it became evident that significant changes had been made that impacted the activity analysis process and the terminology utilized. Thus, a revision of the original *Occupation-Based Activity Analysis* was warranted to offer students and educators a text that reflected the changes made in the *Framework*. This also provided the opportunity to enhance some of the activities, forms, and photos that were in need of improvement. The following is a brief list of some of the major changes made in the second edition:

1. Chapter added: "Determine Relevance and Importance to the Client: Occupation-Based Activity Analysis" to reflect the new addition to the Activity Demands section of the *Framework*.

2. Terminology and definitions changed in Chapter 2 on determining the area of occupation, based on changes in the new *Framework*. Additions and changes have been made to what comprises different occupations.

3. Chapter on body functions reflect changes in terminology and restructuring of what are considered "client factors," which is a significant change in the new *Framework*.

4. The performance skills is the section in the *Framework* that has completely changed, thus the chapter on performance skills is completely revised.

5. The final chapter is focused now on how to utilize aspects of activity analysis for evaluation, intervention planning, and outcomes. This reflects the fact that the new *Framework* considers activity analysis part of the process of occupational therapy, and not the domain. Thus, it is interwoven through all aspects of intervention.

6. Additional activities were provided at the end of each chapter.

7. Appendices and forms have been modified to reflect the changes in the *Framework*.

8. New pictures are included, with greater clarity and resolution.

Additional instructional materials are available to instructors, including PowerPoint presentations for each of the chapters. Please see the SLACK Incorporated website at www.efacultylounge.com for access to these materials.

References

Accreditation Council for Occupational Therapy Education. (2014). *Accreditation Council for Occupational Therapy Education (ACOTE) Standards and Interpretive Guide.*

American Occupational Therapy Association. (2014). Occupational therapy practice framework: Domain and process (3rd ed.). *American Journal of Occupational Therapy, 68*(Suppl. 1):S1-S48.

World Health Organization. (2001). *International classification of functioning, disability, and health.* Geneva, Switzerland: Author.

What Is Activity Analysis?

OBJECTIVES

- Define *activity analysis.*
- Describe the difference between occupation-based activity analysis and activity analysis.
- Identify the current definitions of *occupations.*
- Distinguish between occupations, activities, and tasks.
- Identify why occupational therapy (OT) practitioners utilize occupations and the goals of intervention, as well as the method by which they can reach those goals.
- Describe how activity analysis is utilized by OT practitioners.
- Explain how the *Occupational Therapy Practice Framework 3rd Edition.* (the *Framework*) is utilized as a basis for understanding activity analysis.
- Understand how the *International Classification of Functioning, Disability, and Health* and the World Health Organization (WHO) influence the *Framework.*

- List the steps included in the activity analysis process.

The ability to analyze activities and the occupations in which people engage is fundamental to the practice of OT. Activity analysis is part of the OT process, allowing practitioners to understand and address the skills and external components needed for the performance of any given activity. *Activity analysis* is defined as the process used by OT practitioners that "addresses the typical demands of an activity, the range of skills involved in its performance, and the various cultural meanings that might be ascribed to it" (Crepeau, Cohn, & Boyt Schell, 2003, p. 192). The process of analyzing activities allows the practitioner to understand the demands placed on the person who engages in the activity. A thorough activity analysis will allow for an understanding of the tools and equipment needed; where and with whom the activity takes place; the sequence of steps and timing of those steps; and the body functions, performance skills, and body structures required to perform the activity. Thus, OT professionals learn how to look not only at activities as a whole, but also at their component parts and

Thomas H.
Occupation-Based Activity Analysis, Second Edition (pp 1-11).
© 2015 SLACK Incorporated.

how internal and external contexts contribute to the activities.

Activity analysis has its roots at the very beginnings of our profession. As early as 1917, activity analysis, or *motion study*, was introduced to OT practitioners. Principles guiding how to conduct these analyses were created and published by engineers, establishing methods whereby to study the movements of workers on the job (Gilbreth, 1911; Taylor, 1911). Following this, OT professionals began using these principles to find "what motions are possible or impossible, desirable, or undesirable; then he finds some occupation which involves those possible and desired motions" (Newton, 1919, pp. 4-5). Other professions—such as physical therapy, speech therapy, and engineering—have used these principles in their fields of practice as well.

While analyzing activities may be part of the domain of other professions, for OT practitioners it is essential to the process of OT. The process of OT includes evaluation, intervention, and outcomes. During each of these steps, activity analysis is part of the process. During the evaluation, the OT practitioner must determine the discrepancy between what the client needs or want to do and his or her performance. An OT evaluation begins with an occupational profile, which is an interview with the client. During this interview, the OT gets a fuller picture of what occupations the client is struggling with, the meaning behind those occupations, and in which contexts those occupations occur. This will lead to a list of occupations, each of which will need to be analyzed by the OT to determine the demands of the occupations. The OT will then evaluate the client's performance and use selected assessments to identify and measure specific client factors, skills, or environments. Comparing the demands of the occupation with client performance and environment allows the OT to identify needs. Occupation or activity analysis is an evaluation of the demands of the activity, not an evaluation of the client.

TYPES OF ANALYSES

An activity or occupation-based analysis can be conducted for an individual, a group of individuals (such as a family or group of students), or populations (groups of people living in a specific areas or people who share similar concerns or backgrounds). We have a unique and holistic perspective to activity

analysis as a fundamental component of practice. The OT perspective looks not only at how an activity might be typically done, but also at how it is done and experienced by an individual, examining the internal and external influences on performance and the meaning carried behind the activity. The *Framework* describes two types of activity analysis: (1) activity analysis that looks at the typical demands of an activity and (2) occupation-based activity analysis, which "takes into account the particular person's interests, goals, abilities, and contexts, as well as the demands of the activity itself" (Crepeau, 2003, p. 192). To get a basic understanding of the demands of an activity, without a particular person in mind, you would conduct an activity analysis. If you were analyzing the activity of a specific person, you would conduct an occupation-based activity analysis. Both types of activity analyses are used throughout the process of OT.

To further clarify the difference between an activity analysis and an occupation-based activity analysis, let's take a look at the activity of making a peanut butter and jelly sandwich. We can determine how much range of motion and strength it takes and how much sensory information is required to perform the activity as it might typically be done. However, let's say we go to Lisa's house and analyze how she makes a peanut butter and jelly sandwich for her daughter. The demands of the activity are very different. Her cupboards have child locks on them, which require the use of both hands to open them. The peanut butter she uses for her daughter is extra chunky and is very thick (thus much more difficult to scoop out). Her daughter may be placing extrasensory and attention demands on her (as a 3-year-old often would). Thus, an analysis of the activity demands of Lisa making a peanut butter and jelly sandwich might be better understood as an occupation-based activity analysis (Figure 1-1).

THE ACTIVITY ANALYSIS PROCESS

1. *Activity awareness:* The first part of activity analysis is to establish what you are truly analyzing. Often, activities overlap or become enmeshed in other occupations. Separate the activities into separate and unique activities when possible. From this, you will be able to determine which area of occupation the activity lies in, giving you a fuller picture of what is included in this activity and those surrounding it.

2. You then need to decide what type of analysis you will be conducting. There are essentially two types of activity analysis: (a) occupation-based activity analysis, which is based on a particular client and how he or she engages in the occupation in his or her contexts, and (b) activity analysis of how the activity is typically done, with no particular client in mind. If you are conducting an activity analysis for a client, you will conduct an occupation-based activity analysis; otherwise you will conduct a standard activity analysis. Using either method, the activity or occupation being analyzed must be clearly identified, with specifics that clarify how, where, or in what manner an activity takes place. For instance: "Making a cheese and onion omelet from scratch." For occupation-based activity analysis, this step in the process includes gathering further information about the activity and its relevance and importance to the client. This step is described in full detail in Chapter 3.

3. *Determining the relevance and importance to the client:* This step is included only if you are conducting an occupation-based activity analysis. It requires the practitioner to delve into clients' understanding and definition of their occupations as well as the importance that these occupations have. Gathering this information is the key to successful analysis and the completion of subsequent steps. The ways of collecting this information are presented in Chapter 3.

4. *Identifying the steps required:* This is where you break down the activity into the specific steps and the sequence and timing of each step. By listing the steps required by the activity, the practitioner is able to identify the demands of the activity. This process is explained in detail in Chapter 4.

5. *Determining the objects and properties:* Considering each of the steps of the activity, specific tools, supplies, and equipment may be needed. Identifying the needed objects allows the practitioner to understand what must be manipulated or interacted with and how. An understanding of the objects and their properties may also lead the practitioner to understand deficits in performance. This is described in Chapter 5.

6. *Determining the space demands:* The physical environment in which an activity or occupation take place can have a great impact on performance. Some activities require specific space, noise control, and lighting in order to be engaged in. There may be times when the physical environment in

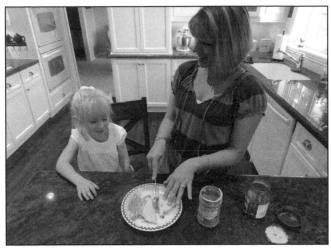

Figure 1-1. Lisa making a sandwich as an occupation.

which an occupation takes place may be a barrier to a client's performance. It is in understanding the physical environment in which an activity takes place that we can view how external forces play a role in occupational performance. This is also described in Chapter 5.

7. *Determining social demands:* Just as space demands can be an external influence on performance, so too can social demands. Social demands of some activities are a necessary part of engaging in an activity (such as taking turns in a game). However, in some occupations, the social demands may challenge the client to a greater extent than he or she is able to manage (e.g., expectations from others to work 16-hour days). The process of determining the social demands of an activity is described in Chapter 5.

8. *Determining required body functions:* This step in the analysis process is often seen as the most detailed and extensive. Many of the concepts parallel those used in other professions. However, the OT activity analysis process goes further. Body functions are those "physiological functions of body systems" (WHO, 2001, p. 10) that include not just physical functions such as strength and mobility of joints, but also sensory, cognitive, and emotional functions. Determining the body functions required of an activity provides information regarding what is demanded of the client in regard to engagement in the occupation or activity. The body functions are described in detail in Chapter 6.

9. *Determining required body structures:* Most activities require the presence of certain body structures.

TABLE 1-1
CASE EXAMPLE: TRAVIS
Step 1: Define the activity: What are we going to analyze? What meaning lies behind the activities and what defines success? Decide on how you would divide the parts of his job so that you could analyze them accurately (see Chapter 2).
Step 2: List the steps of the activity: Write out the steps Travis must follow in order to successfully complete each activity or task. You may have several lists, one for each activity (see Chapter 3).
Step 3: Define the objects, properties, space, and social demands: What are the objects, materials, and equipment that Travis must use (see Chapter 4)?
Step 4: Define the space demands: What are the environmental requirements for the activity to be performed successfully (see Chapter 5)?
Step 5: Define the social demands: What are the social rules or expectations of the activity (see Chapter 5)?
Step 6: Define the required body functions: What mental, physical, neurological, and other body functions are utilized and challenged during the activities that Travis must perform (see Chapter 5)?
Step 7: List the required body structures: What parts of the body are required to complete the activities (see Chapter 6)?
Step 8: Define the performance skills: What motor, praxis, sensory, emotional, cognitive, and communication/social skill levels are needed to complete the activities (see Chapter 7)?

Body structures are "anatomical parts of the body such as organs, limbs, and their components" (WHO, 2001, p.10). In the activity analysis process, we look at which body structures are required for the activity beyond what is required for sustaining life. This is described further in Chapter 7.

10. *Determining required performance skills:* Performance skills are actions that the client demonstrates. Determining the level of specific skills required allows the practitioner to better understand what is expected from the client for successful engagement. The performance skills are explained in detail in Chapter 8.

11. *Analyzing for therapeutic intervention:* This is the step of the process in which the practitioner evaluates an activity as well as the needs of the client so as to find possible outcomes. An activity can also be analyzed in order to find ways to adapt or grade the activity to either decrease or increase the challenge for the client. This is be explained in detail in Chapter 9.

To better understand how this process works, let's take a look at a real case example (Table 1-1). Travis is a 31-year-old male who was injured on the job 2 months earlier when he hit his head on a large piece of machinery and lost consciousness. He works at a factory that makes and packages potato chips. Travis works on an assembly line, putting small bags of potato chips into variety-pack boxes. He has come to OT to receive a return-to-work assessment. To do this, we will use our activity analysis skills. Because this is an activity analysis for a specific client, we will be conducting an occupation-based activity analysis.

To begin the analysis, we interview Travis and he tells us about his job and what his job entails. We then separate the different activities that he described, which are part of his job. During the interview, Travis defines each activity, delineating what success means in each. We begin with one activity, listing each step. The next step is to evaluate what objects are needed and the properties of each of these objects. Next, we look at the space and social demands that Travis has in the work setting for the activity. We then analyze what body functions and structures are needed for him to do the activity. The final step requires that we identify which performance skills are required and to what extent.

Once the activity analysis is complete, a full evaluation of Travis' performance and abilities will need to be conducted.

After these steps, you will be able to develop an intervention plan and make recommendations for adaptations that will hopefully allow Travis to return to work.

WHAT ARE OCCUPATIONS VERSUS ACTIVITIES?

The term *occupation* can often be misunderstood and may be misleading. If you were to ask someone off the street, perhaps someone without a medical background, what his or her occupation was, he or she would probably begin to tell you about the jobs he or she has had in the past. As a student, you may have already had the experience of trying to tell family members and friends what you will be studying and that "No, it's not about helping people get jobs." *Merriam-Webster's Collegiate Dictionary* (2012) defines *occupation* in several ways:

1. An activity in which one engages
2. The principle business of one's life: vocation
3. The possession, use, or settlement of land: occupancy
4. The holding and control of an area by a foreign military force

Thus, it is understandable that when people hear the term *occupation* in respect to therapy, numerous configurations of this profession may come to mind. This also explains why some countries use a term other than *occupation* to describe our profession (Box 1-1). However, medical dictionaries define the term *occupation* in a much broader, yet personal, way. In *Taber's Cyclopedic Medical Dictionary*, Venes (2001) defines *occupation* as follows:

1. Any goal-directed pursuit in which one works for a wage, salary, or other income
2. Any goal-directed use of time
3. Any activity or pursuit in which one is engaged outside of one's work

The second and third definitions listed better match how health care professionals, including OT professionals, understand the term. Scholars of OT have defined *occupation* in several ways:

> Occupation is used to mean all the things people want, need, or have to do, whether of physical, mental, social, sexual, political, or spiritual nature and is inclusive of sleep and

---

Box 1-1

The term *occupation* is not used to describe our profession in some countries, where terms that stem from the ideas of ergonomics or recovery are used. The following are a few examples of what occupational therapy is called in other countries:

Austria:	*Ergotherapie*
Belgium:	*L'ergothérapeute*
Finland:	*Toimintaterapia*
India:	*Ergomedicine*
Malaysia:	*Pemulihan Cara Kerja*
Sweden:	*Arbeitsterapeuter*

Adapted from World Federation of Occupational Therapy. (2009-2010). Definitions of occupational therapy from member countries, draft 9. Retrieved from http://www.wfot.org/resourcecentre.aspx

---

rest. It refers to all aspects of actual human doing, being, becoming, and belonging. The practical, everyday medium of self-expression or of making or experiencing meaning, occupation is the activist element of human existence whether occupations are contemplative, reflective, and meditative or action based. (Wilcock & Townsend, 2014, p. 542)

> Activities … of everyday life, named, organized, and given value and meaning by individuals and a culture. Occupation is everything people do to occupy themselves, including looking after themselves … enjoying life … and contributing to the social and economic fabric of their communities. (Law, Polatajko, Baptiste, & Townsend, 1997, p. 32)

> Goal-directed pursuits that typically extend over time, have meaning to the performance, and involve multiple tasks. (Christiansen et al., 2005, p. 548)

> The things that people do that occupy their time and attention; meaningful, purposeful activity; the personal activities that individuals chose or need to engage in and the ways in which each individual actually experiences them. (Boyt Schell, Gillen, & Scaffa, 2014, p. 1237)

Given these definitions, occupations are more than just activities; they are the activities that give our lives meaning. Many articles have been written and discussions conducted on the differences between

ACTIVITY 1-1

Take a second to think about the occupations in which you engage. List a few of them below. Then ask yourself: Has each one met the four criteria of an occupation as described by Carlson and Clark?

OCCUPATION	START AND END	INTENTIONAL AND REPEATABLE	MEANINGFUL	LABELED BY CULTURE

occupations, activities, and tasks (Gray, 1998; Nelson, 1988; Pierce, 2001; Trombly, 1995). Many authors agree that occupations comprise a greater, more personalized definition of activities, within which smaller tasks lie (Law et al., 1997; Trombly, 1995). The *Framework* identifies occupations as including multiple activities. Occupations occur within the context of a person or group, having unique purpose and meaning to the person engaging in a given occupation. Contexts include the physical environment, the tools and materials that the person uses, and the social complexities and demands of the occupation. Thus, occupations are "personalized" activities—those that hold personal meaning and requirements for a particular person or group. An occupation is much more complex than an activity.

To give further clarity to the domain of our practice of occupations, Larson, Wood, and Clark (2003) have delineated how occupations differ from activities:

There are definitive start and end points. The participant can choose to begin and to end.

Activity: Making a peanut butter and jelly sandwich.

Occupation: Lisa making a peanut butter and jelly sandwich for her daughter at home.

Tasks: Taking a plate out of the cupboard, getting the peanut butter out of the refrigerator, etc.

Occupations are intentionally executed and repeatable, such that something that is outside of the person's control of repeating, such as an illness or accident, are not considered occupations.

Occupations are meaningful to the person and bring meaning to who they are as a person. This meaning may be fairly insignificant, or even unhealthy (smoking, for example), yet they still play a part in the meaning of the person's life.

Occupations are labeled by our culture. New occupations are created every day, and the occupations people engage in change over time.

The profession of OT views occupations not only as the ends of our interventions, but also as the means by which we reach those goals. Thus, it is important to understand the depth of how much more *occupation* means vs *activity* (Activity 1-1).

WHY OCCUPATIONS?

We now understand that our goal is to be able to analyze the activities that bring meaning to our clients' lives—which we call occupations. But why do we need to analyze these occupations? We use occupations (and activities) not only as our goals, but also as the means by which we meet those goals; thus, occupations and activities are our "tools." No other profession

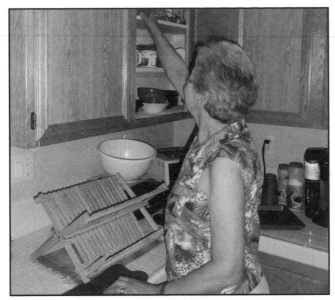

Figure 1-2. Kay gaining mastery of occupations in the kitchen.

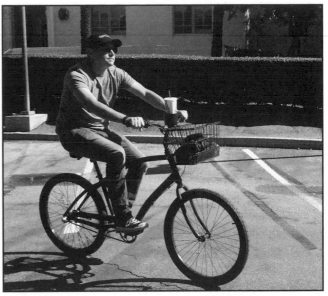

Figure 1-3. Occupations encourage greater and longer engagement.

can claim to use occupations as a therapeutic modality, as we do. We use occupations or meaningful activities as interventions because we understand the greater benefit of using activities that are meaningful versus other techniques or approaches. The benefits or rewards are often hidden behind the "normalcy" of everyday activities. The following are just some of the many benefits of using occupations as the center of our interventions:

- Engaging in occupations allows clients to achieve mastery in the environment. It allows them to feel that they have some sense of control. For example, if our client Kay does overhead reaching exercises using a dowel, she may build up her shoulder strength to eventually reach into her cupboards. However, if you have her actually move cups from a lower position, up into cupboards, she will not only build up shoulder strength, but also learn strategies for how she can continue to do this at home, thus gaining a sense of mastery over being able to utilize her kitchen again (Figure 1-2).

- Engaging in occupations often results in something that the client can either see or feel. The result may be a tangible object (although many times it is not) or the result may be something the client can feel. Using the example of putting cups away in the cupboard, Kay can see the results of her efforts; the cups are put away in the cupboard and she feels a sense of accomplishment. Participating in an occupation can result in a sense of accomplishment.

- Engaging in a meaningful activity will often help the client go farther and longer toward a goal than other methods. If the attention is on the goal or the enjoyment of the process, then the client may become "engaged" and lost in participating in the activity. For example, when I go to the gym, I will often try to ride the stationary bike. In the cold, boring gym, I can usually last about 15 minutes before calling it quits. However, if I get on my bike at home and ride around the neighborhood, I can ride for hours. Why? The bike ride around my neighborhood is a more meaningful activity to me (Figure 1-3). *"Occupations encourage greater and longer engagement."* I get lost and occupied in the surroundings and variety. While both are very similar and provide the same physical challenges, one will end up with a greater result, simply because it is able to get me "engaged" in it.

- Occupations allow for greater transference toward the client's goals. Intervention that engages the client in occupations or parts of the greater occupation ensures that the intervention time will lead to application toward the goal. For example, let's say you have your client Lance spend a lot of time in therapy picking up beans and putting them in a cup. However, when it comes time for Lance to be able to pick up and take his own medications, there is no guarantee that the time picking up beans will have helped. This is often termed *generalization*. Can clients generalize what you are doing with them or during therapy to the real world? For many clients with cognitive deficits, this is very difficult. Thus, using activities that are closer to the clients' desired occupations helps to ensure that they will be able to apply what they have learned or gained to their own lives.

- Engaging in occupations requires a coordination of different skills and body systems. To help clarify this point, let's take another look at Kay's ability to put dishes away in her cupboards. One treatment strategy to help her reach the goal of putting dishes away might be to have her do upper extremity exercises. During these, she utilizes her upper body strength, range of motion, proprioception, and ability to follow directions. However, if we have her actually put cups in a cupboard, she will be working on upper body strength; range of motion; proprioception; and the skills of stabilization, reaching, coordination, manipulation, grip, handling objects, sequencing, spatial organization, and accommodation of movements. Kay is not just working on one skill or client factor in isolation, but rather on many together, learning how to use all of them to accomplish the task.

- By engaging in occupations, the client receives immediate feedback on performance. Feedback on performance can come from the task itself, the therapist, or the clients themselves. For example, say Kay is trying to reach up and put a cup on a shelf. She is struggling and not quite able to reach. The therapist can give her feedback and suggestions, such as, "Step closer to the shelf," or encouragement, such as, "You are almost there." But Kay is also getting visual feedback by seeing how far away she is from the goal of reaching the shelf, and she receives feedback from her body on how it feels to reach that high. Perhaps her shoulder is weak or becomes painful when she is reaching. This is all feedback that is immediate and directly related to her goal.

WHY DO WE LEARN TO ANALYZE ACTIVITIES AND OCCUPATIONS?

Being able to analyze the meaningful activities (the occupations) of our clients' lives is essential to every aspect of our practice. The *Framework* is a fundamental document published by the American Occupational Therapy Association (AOTA) that describes the domain and process within which OT occurs. In this document, the OT process is described as involving evaluation, intervention, and outcomes (AOTA, 2014). The ability to examine and analyze the activities that are important to the client is essential in all steps, especially in evaluation and intervention. The analysis of activities becomes instinctive and second nature to seasoned practitioners, as it is a part of understanding each client, establishing goals, creating interventions, and determining outcomes. The information from an activity analysis provides essential information in the following ways:

- It identifies needed equipment, materials, space, and time.
- It provides a knowledge base for instructing others by outlining each step and how it is done.
- It gives information on how an activity might be therapeutic and for whom.
- It helps to grade or adapt the activity to allow for greater success.
- It gives specifics for clear documentation.
- It assists in discovering how contexts influence the performance of an occupation.
- It helps to select appropriate activities and find the "just-right challenge."
- It identifies areas in which the client needs help and intervention.

Thus, we begin our journey with our clients by analyzing their activities and looking carefully at the details of the occupations they wish to engage in and what defines *success* in the performance of these occupations. This includes being able to analyze all of the demands of the activity for that person in his or her contexts. In order to create challenging intervention strategies, activities are analyzed to find their therapeutic benefit. The steps and requirements of the activity may be teased apart in order to adapt the activity. Before working with a client, therapists will often mentally analyze multiple activities in order to find the ideal challenge for the client during the coming session. The analyses often continue during the session as the therapist watches a client struggle or succeed, and the activity may need to be adapted or graded to allow for greater challenges or successes. At the time of reevaluation or assessment of outcomes, the therapist must once again analyze the client's activities and occupations in order to establish what defines success for that client in his or her contexts. The occupational therapist, as an expert at everyday activity, utilizes his or her expertise in activity analysis throughout practice.

THE OCCUPATIONAL THERAPY PRACTICE FRAMEWORK, 3RD EDITION: THE BASIS FOR ACTIVITY ANALYSIS

Mentioned earlier in this chapter, the *Framework* is the basis on which this text was developed. Therefore, it should be explained why and how this document was established. Previous to the establishment of the *Framework*, the document guiding OT terminology was the *Universal Terminology III* (UT-III), published by the AOTA in 1994 (AOTA, 2014). Since then, the profession has evolved and grown. Much of the language used in the UT-III was exclusively used by OT practitioners and was not recognized by other professions. A committee was developed in 1998 to begin revising this document. This committee decided that instead of revising a document that only defined terminology, they would develop a new document that would not only establish terminology but also define and clarify the domain of our professional practice. The UT-III was rescinded and a new document was created, using the WHO's *International Classification of Functioning, Disability, and Health* (ICF) as a guide.

The WHO is the leader and coordinator of global health-related issues within the United Nations. This organization directs research agendas, sets standards and norms, and studies health trends on a global level (WHO, 2001). The ICF is a document that was created by the WHO as a framework for classifying health and disability. It redefined for many what was thought of as disability, recognizing that disability has a social aspect and is not always a biological disorder but can be a result of socioeconomic or environmental factors as well. Another purpose of the ICF is to provide a common language and terminology for health professionals internationally and across multiple disciplines. This document is available publicly through the WHO website (www.who.int/en).

By using the terminology and classifications used in the ICF, the language used in the *Framework* is internationally and interprofessionally recognized. The first edition of the *Framework* was created by the AOTA's Commission on Practice and was published in 2002 (AOTA, 2014). The *Framework* was created as a document that would serve to "define and guide occupational therapy practice" (AOTA, 2008, p. 625). As the profession continued to grow and progress, the AOTA published the second edition in 2008 and the third edition in 2014, with each revision refining and enhancing the original document as the profession continued to evolve and grow.

The *Framework* did more than define terminology for the profession of OT by establishing a clear definition of our domain and the process in which OT practice occurs. What is our focus when we work with a client? How are we different from other disciplines? If "everyday life activity" is our focus, what does that mean? The *Framework* demonstrates the complexity of everyday activities and how each component works together to allow for participation in meaningful activities. In describing the focus of practice, it also provides a foundation for activity analysis and will thus be the basis on which we analyze activities and occupations in this book (Table 1-2).

CONCLUSION

The ability to analyze activities and occupations is a skill essential to the practice of OT. OT practitioners have a unique view of what comprises daily activities and what contributes to a person's engagement in an activity. Our focus is not simply on activities, but on meaningful activities that are part of people's lives—occupations. Occupations are the focus of our profession, not only as a goal for our clients, but also as the means by which we help them meet those goals. Thus, it is important to understand all of the elements that contribute to a person's ability to participate in the occupations that are meaningful to him or her. Using the activity demands section of the *Framework* as a basis on which to analyze occupations and activities allows the clinician to gain a full understanding of what aspects should be included in an analysis. The steps to activity analysis listed earlier in this chapter are explained in greater detail in the chapters following, walking the reader through the process of activity analysis.

QUESTIONS

1. How are occupations different than activities?
2. In what ways are occupations used in OT practice?
3. Why do OT practitioners use occupations during intervention?

TABLE 1-2
ACTIVITY DEMANDS

Relevance and importance to client: Client's goals, values, beliefs, needs, and perceived utility.
Objects and their properties: The tools, supplies, and equipment used in the process of carrying out the activity.
Space demands: The physical environment requirements of the activity.
Social demands: The social environment, virtual environment, and cultural contexts that may be required by the activity.
Sequence and timing: The process used to carry out the activity (specific steps, sequence, timing requirements).
Required actions: The usual skills that would be required by any performer to carry out the activity. Sensory, perceptual, motor, praxis, emotional, cognitive, communication, and social performance skills should each be considered. The performance skills demanded by an activity will be correlated with the demands of the other activity aspects (i.e., objects, space).
Required body functions: "Physiological functions of body systems (including psychological functions)" (WHO, 2001, p. 10) that are required to support the actions used to perform the activity.
Required body structures: "Anatomical parts of the body such as organs, limbs, and their components (that support body function)" (WHO, 2001, p. 10) that are required to perform the activity.
Adapted from American Occupational Therapy Association. (2014). Occupational therapy practice framework: Domain and process (3rd ed.). *American Journal of Occupational Therapy, 68*(Suppl. 1), S1-S48. Retrieved from http://dx.doi.org/10.5014/ajot.2014.682006

4. What does conducting an activity analysis provide for the practitioner? How does it help with the intervention process?

5. What are the basic steps of an activity analysis?

6. Read the *Occupational Therapy Practice Framework, 3rd Edition.* Why is this document used to guide the activity analysis process?

ACTIVITIES

1. Look up the ICF on the WHO website. How does the ICF define *disability*?

2. Interview an OT practitioner. Ask how he or she utilizes activity analysis in everyday practice.

3. Create a visual representation of the steps required for activity analysis. Use a variety of objects and materials to represent this process.

REFERENCES

American Occupational Therapy Association. (2008). Occupational therapy practice framework: Domain and process (2nd ed.). *American Journal of Occupational Therapy, 62*(6), 609-639.

American Occupational Therapy Association. (2014). Occupational therapy practice framework: Domain and process (3rd ed.). *American Journal of Occupational Therapy, 68*(Suppl. 1), S1-S48. Retrieved from http://dx.doi.org/10.5014/ajot.2014.682006

Boyt Schell, B. A., Gillen, G., & Scaffa, M. (2014). Glossary. In B. A. Boyt Schell, G. Gillen, & M. Scaffa (Eds.). *Willard and Spackman's occupational therapy* (12th ed., pp. 1229-1243). Philadelphia, PA: Lippincott Williams & Wilkins.

Christiansen, C., Baum, C. M., & Bass-Haugen, J. (Eds.) (2005). *Occupational therapy: Performance, participation, and well-being.* Thorofare, NJ: SLACK Incorporated.

Crepeau, E. (2003). Analyzing occupation and activity: A way of thinking about occupational performance: In E. Crepeau, E. Cohn, & B.A. Boyt Schell (Eds.). *Willard and Spackman's occupational therapy* (10th ed., pp. 189-198). Philadelphia, PA: Lippincott Williams & Wilkins.

Crepeau, E., Cohn, E., & Boyt Schell, B. A. (Eds.). (2003). *Willard & Spackman's occupational therapy* (10th ed.). Philadelphia, PA: Lippincott Williams & Wilkins.

Gilbreth, F. B. (1911). *Motion study.* New York, NY: Van Nostrand.

Gray, J. M. (1998). Putting occupation into practice: Occupation as ends, occupation as means. *American Journal of Occupational Therapy, 52,* 354-364.

Larson, E., Wood, W., & Clark, F. (2003). Occupational science: Building the science and practice of occupation through an academic discipline. In E. Crepeau, E. Cohn, & B. Boyt Schell, (Eds.). *Willard and Spackman's occupational therapy* (10th ed., pp. 15-26). Philadelphia, PA: Lippincott Williams & Wilkins.

Law, M., Polatajko, H., Baptiste, W., & Townsend, E. (1997). Core concepts of occupational therapy. In E. Townsend (Ed.), *Enabling occupation: An occupational therapy perspective* (pp. 29-56). Ottawa, ON: Canadian Association of Occupational Therapists.

Merriam-Webster, Inc. (2012). *Merriam-Webster's collegiate dictionary* (11th ed). Springfield, MA: Merriam-Webster, Inc.

Nelson, D. L. (1988). Occupation: Form and function. *American Journal of Occupational Therapy, 42,* 633-642.

Newton, I. G. (1919). *Consolation house.* Clifton Springs, NY: Consolation House.

Pierce, D. (2001). Untangling occupation and activity. *American Journal of Occupational Therapy, 55,* 138-146.

Taylor, F. W. (1911). *The principles of scientific management.* New York, NY: Harper & Brothers.

Trombly, C. A. (1995). Occupation, purposefulness and meaningfulness as therapeutic mechanisms [Eleanor Clark Slagle Lecture]. *American Journal of Occupational Therapy, 49,* 960-972.

Venes, D. (Ed.). (2001). *Taber's cyclopedic medical dictionary* (19th ed.). Philadelphia, PA: F.A. Davis Company.

Wilcock, A. A., & Townsend, E. A. (2014). Occupational justice. In B. A. Boyt Schell, G. Gillen, & M. Scaffa (Eds.). *Willard and Spackman's occupational therapy* (12th ed., pp. 541-552). Philadelphia, PA: Lippincott Williams & Wilkins.

World Health Organization. (2001). *International classification of functioning, disability, and health.* Geneva, Switzerland: Author.

STEPS TO ACTIVITY ANALYSIS

Step 1: Determine What Is Being Analyzed
Chapter 2

Step 2: Determine the Relevance
and Importance to the Client
Chapter 3

Step 3: Determine the Sequence and Timing
Chapter 4

Step 4: Determine Object, Space,
and Social Demands
Chapter 5

Step 5: Determine Required Body Functions
Chapter 6

Step 6: Determine Required Body Structures
Chapter 7

Step 7: Determine Required Actions
and Performance Skills
Chapter 8

2

Step 1: Determine What Is Being Analyzed

OBJECTIVES

- Understand how an occupation-based activity analysis is different from a standard activity analysis.
- Determine when to conduct an occupation-based activity analysis or a standard activity analysis.
- Divide a large occupation into smaller manageable activities or tasks to allow for analysis.
- Understand why the *Occupational Therapy Practice Framework, 3rd Edition* (the *Framework*) has classified and defined occupations into separate areas.
- Define the types and categories of occupations listed in the *Framework*.
- Understand how each area of occupation relates to occupational therapy (OT) practice.
- Identify the difference between activities of daily living (ADL), instrumental activities of daily living (IADL), rest and sleep, work, education, play, leisure, and social participation.

- Understand how occupations can be classified in different areas of occupation based on the client.

OCCUPATION-BASED OR STANDARD ACTIVITY ANALYSIS?

The first step to activity analysis is to determine what it is that you will be analyzing. As discussed in Chapter 1, there are two types of activity analysis: activity analysis and occupation-based activity analysis. The first type, activity analysis, involves analyzing an activity as it is typically done, without a particular person in mind. This is helpful when looking at different activities and how they might be therapeutic. Occupation-based activity analysis is very individualized, as it looks at an activity that has meaning and contextual influences for a particular individual. Going back to the example of making a peanut butter and jelly sandwich, an activity analysis could be completed on how it is typically done, but an occupation-based activity analysis would be completed if we looked at how Lisa does it.

Thomas H.
Occupation-Based Activity Analysis, Second Edition (pp 13-42).
© 2015 SLACK Incorporated.

ACTIVITY 2-1

Using the definition of an occupation (see Chapter 1), determine if the following activities would require an activity analysis or an occupation-based activity analysis.

ACTIVITY	ACTIVITY ANALYSIS	OCCUPATION-BASED ACTIVITY ANALYSIS
Putting pegs into a pegboard		
How to sew a button on a shirt		
How a client will make tea		
Riding a bike		
Mary putting dishes into her dishwasher		
Mary stacking cones on the table		
Writing a paper for an OT class		

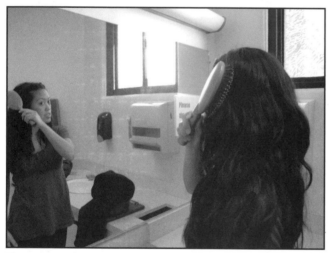

Figure 2-1. Task: styling hair.

The first step to your analysis is to determine if you will be conducting an occupation-based activity analysis or just an activity analysis. Both are done within the process of OT evaluation and intervention (Activity 2-1).

NARROWING DOWN THE ACTIVITY OR OCCUPATION TO BE ANALYZED

After you have determined this, you must then determine what specific activity or occupation you will be analyzing. If it is too large, it needs to be broken down into smaller activities or tasks. Some authors believe

that occupations are made up of smaller "tasks" (Hagedorn, 1995, 1997). For example, if you were to look at the larger occupation of snow skiing, this occupation is made up of several activities or tasks, such as putting on the gear, buying a lift ticket, getting onto the ski lift, and then skiing down the hill. Each of these contributes to participation in snow skiing and can be analyzed from an activity or occupation-based activity analysis standpoint. For many occupations and activities, breaking it down into smaller tasks is a necessary step. To decide whether this is necessary, think about the following:

- Are there more than 10 to 15 steps? If so, break the activity up into separate activities to analyze. For example, putting on pants and putting on underwear can be separated.

- Are there multiple criteria for successful completion? For example, perhaps getting dressed includes getting pants, shirt, socks, and shoes on correctly. Instead of analyzing "getting dressed" perhaps analyzing "putting on a shirt" and each other task would be more effective.

- Are there different objects or space demands for different parts of the activity? For example, if you were to analyze "getting ready in the morning," there are parts of the activity that require the use of the bedroom (obtaining and donning clothes), as well as the use of the bathroom (showering, brushing teeth). There are also very different objects required for parts of this activity. Towels, soap, and shampoo are required for showering, while a comb or brush is required for the grooming part of getting ready in the morning (Figure 2-1). Finding that

---

ACTIVITY 2-2

Take a moment to think about each of the following activities. How would you break them down into smaller tasks, or would you analyze them as they are? If the activity listed cannot be broken down any further, check off the box that states "Keep As Is."

ACTIVITY	KEEP AS IS	SEPARATE ACTIVITIES
Washing a car		
Sewing a button on a shirt		
Cleaning the kitchen		
Making scrambled eggs		
Gardening		
Taking care of cats		

---

there are very distinct groupings of objects and settings might signal to you that the activity needs to be broken down into smaller tasks. In this example, the activity of getting ready in the morning can be broken down into tasks such as showering, brushing teeth, using the toilet, and combing and styling hair (Activity 2-2).

IDENTIFYING THE OCCUPATION

The domain of our practice is occupations or the everyday activities that make up people's lives (AOTA, 2014). This means all activities that people may engage in are of concern to us. The *Framework* helps to define what this means by listing all human activities in categories called areas of occupation. The most common life activities are categorized into eight areas: ADL, IADL, rest and sleep, education, work, play, leisure, and social participation. Under each of these areas are categories describing common activities for that area of occupation, followed by a list of activities that might fall under that category. For example, bathing and showering are one of the categories under the ADL area of occupation. Activities included in bathing and showering are "obtaining supplies; soaping, rinsing, and drying body parts; maintaining bathing position; and transferring to and from bathing positions" (AOTA, 2014, p. S19).

The range of different occupations is found in Table 1 of the *Framework*. They broadly define all occupations and give the reader an idea of the breadth of the scope of OT. Using this classification system helps OT practitioners in many ways.

It clarifies the scope of our practice, not only for occupational therapists and occupational therapy assistants (OTAs), but also for other health care professionals and consumers. By defining all areas of occupation, everyone understands what areas we address. It exemplifies that we are more than the ADL or self-care experts but rather that we look at all activities that are meaningful in people's lives.

It is a cue for occupational therapists and OTAs as to all of the areas we are responsible for. If I was injured in a car accident and needed the services of OT, I would want the professionals working with me to recognize all areas of my life that are important. It is important not only that I be able to dress myself and take myself to the bathroom, but also that I be able to socially participate in family gatherings, engage in leisure activities, and take care of my cats. This list of occupations is often an eye-opener for students as they see the extent of what our profession entails. Yes, sexual activity and sleep are also occupations that are part of our domain!

Each category of an occupation gives examples of the activities and tasks that make up that area of occupation. The complexity of everyday activities is often overlooked. Listing the multiple tasks that are required of occupations illustrates how multifaceted some of these everyday activities are.

The terminology of the areas of occupation and their categories helps practitioners use universal language in their documentation. The *Framework* was created using language from the World Health

Organization's *International Classification of Functioning, Disability, and Health* (WHO, 2001); thus, the terminology is internationally and interprofessionally recognized. The use of this language to document and discuss your client's occupations will ensure greater understanding by other health care professionals, as well as funding sources.

Understanding what defines each area of occupation helps us determine what we need to assess and evaluate in our clients. What does it mean to be independent in ADL? Using the list of occupations the *Framework* provides as a guide, we know all of the tasks and activities this entails. If I were to watch my client, Jennifer, get dressed and complete her grooming independently, could I say that she is independent in all of her ADL? What about bathing, bowel and bladder management, eating, feeding, functional mobility, personal device care, toilet hygiene, and the other activities listed as ADL in the *Framework*? Of course, we must only consider all of the ADL that Jennifer considers important and a part of her life. For example, "personal device care" is a subcategory of the ADL area of occupation. This includes the care and use of personal items such as hearing aids, contact lenses, glasses, orthotic or prosthetic devices, adaptive equipment, and contraceptive or sexual devices. Perhaps Jennifer does not use any personal devices. Would we consider this as part of her ADL? We would not, unless she were to begin using such a device soon, like a prosthetic or orthotic device.

THE AREAS OF OCCUPATION

Activities of Daily Living

"Activities that are oriented toward taking care of one's own body" (AOTA, 2014, p. S19).

This area of occupation is often the first thing people think of when they think of OT. ADL are the basic self-care skills required for daily living. Christiansen and Hammecker (2001) believe that the ADL activities are "fundamental to living in a social world; they enable basic survival and well-being" (p. 156). Activities such as eating and bowel and bladder management are examples of ADL that are essential to survival, not to mention maintaining health. These activities are often part of the routines built into our daily lives. A

decline in this area is often the first sign of disease or illness (Rogers & Holm, 1994).

ADL are often called personal activities of daily living, and for good reason: many of the activities are very personal or have to do with care of the body. For example, requiring assistance with tasks such as cleaning and wiping the body after using the toilet may be seen as embarrassing and difficult to accept. Thus, independence in these private areas of self-care often becomes a priority. As you review each of these areas, think about how important it is to you that you be able to do these things for yourself.

Bathing and Showering

"Obtaining and using supplies; soaping, rinsing, and drying body parts; maintaining bathing position; and transferring to and from bathing positions" (AOTA, 2014, p. S19).

This defines bathing, which can be done in a tub, shower, bed, sink, or other setting, while sitting, standing, or lying down. The *Framework* does not specify that bathing or showering must be completed in a particular environment or with specific equipment or objects, but it does specify the tasks that the person should complete in order to bathe the body. The first task is obtaining all supplies, including towels, soap, shampoo, or whatever the individual client requires for safe and complete cleaning of the body. The client must soap the entire body, rinse the soap off, and dry all body parts. While bathing, the client must maintain the position and move to and from bathing positions needed to clean all areas of the body. Let's go back to our client, Jennifer, to better understand this. Let's say she is going to bathe in a shower using a shower chair. She needs to be able to get into the shower (this can be done in many ways), sit down on the shower chair, and shift her weight and move into different positions so that she can clean all areas of her body without losing her balance and falling. She also needs to be able to get out of the shower safely.

Toileting and Toilet Hygiene

"Obtaining and using toileting supplies; clothing management; maintaining toileting position; transferring to and from toileting position; cleaning body; and caring for menstrual and continence needs (including catheters, colostomies, and suppository management) as well as

completing intentional control of bowel movements and urinary bladder and, if necessary, using equipment or agents for bladder control" (AOTA, 2014, p. S19).

Toileting includes both the use of toileting objects and managing clothing and cleaning oneself; it also includes bowel and bladder management. This consists of emptying the bowel or the bladder and may include the use of devices or medical agents—such as catheters, rectal stimulators, and suppositories—in order to complete those tasks. Let's use Juanita as an example to define toilet hygiene. Juanita has a spinal cord injury and no longer has control over her bowels or bladder. In order to empty her bladder, Juanita must move forward to the edge of her wheelchair, where she then lowers her pants to her knees. She then uses a urinary catheter, disposes of the urine and catheter, cleans herself, and then pulls up her pants and scoots back into her wheelchair. These are all elements of toileting and toilet hygiene for Juanita.

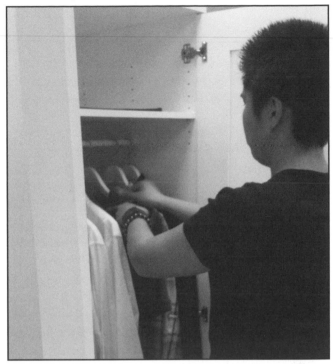

Figure 2-2. Dressing includes selecting appropriate clothing.

Dressing

"Selecting clothing and accessories appropriate to time of day, weather, and occasion; obtaining clothing from storage area; dressing and undressing in a sequential fashion; fastening and adjusting clothing and shoes; and applying and removing personal devices, prosthetic devices, or splints" (AOTA, 2014, p. S19).

This explains that dressing is not only about donning (putting on) and doffing (taking off) clothing. Dressing includes being able to pick out clothing that is appropriate for the weather and the situation the person is going to be in. Once the person has chosen what he or she wants, it will also be necessary to remove the clothing from the storage area, such as a closet (Figure 2-2), drawer, or laundry basket. Once the clothing items have been obtained, they need to be put on in the correct order (the underpants cannot be put on after the pants), and all zippers, ties, buttons, buckles, and Velcro must be fastened. This applies not only to putting on clothing items, but also taking them off. Prosthetic and orthotic devices are also part of the body and are thus also included in dressing. An orthotic device, such as a splint, is designed to control or correct a bony deformity or lack of strength or control of a part of the body (Deshaies, 2008). Hand splints, ankle supports, and back braces are examples of orthotics. Prosthetics are devices that replace a limb or body function. Examples are artificial legs, arms, and hands and hearing aids. Therefore, while orthotics help support, control, or correct, prosthetics actually replace body functions.

Swallowing/Eating

"Keeping and manipulating food or fluid in the mouth and swallowing it; swallowing is moving food from the mouth to the stomach" (AOTA, 2014, p. S19).

Feeding

"The process of setting up, arranging, and bringing food [or fluid] from the plate or cup to the mouth; sometimes called self-feeding" (AOTA, 2014, p. S19).

The terms *eating* and *feeding* are often misunderstood and used interchangeably, which is incorrect. Feeding includes the tasks that occur from the plate to the mouth, and eating/swallowing includes the tasks that follow, once the food reaches the mouth. It makes more sense if you think of the two in context. Imagine that you are lying on a beach somewhere relaxing. Some attractive man or woman (you fill in your own fantasy) is feeding you grapes. He or she

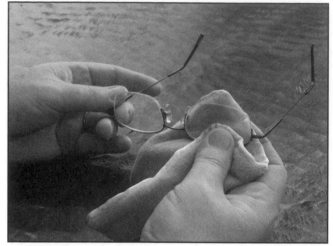

Figure 2-3. Cleaning eyeglasses is an example of personal device care.

picks the grapes off of a bunch and brings them to your mouth. You then eat the grapes by chewing them, moving them around your mouth, and swallowing them. Thus, eating and feeding occur together but are different activities and require very different skills. A right-handed person with a spinal injury leaving his right side paralyzed may have difficulty with feeding but not eating. His ability or lack of ability to move his right hand has no influence on his ability to chew and swallow.

Functional Mobility

"Moving from one position or place to another (during performance of everyday activities), such as in-bed mobility, wheelchair mobility, transfers (wheelchair, bed, car, tub, toilet, tub/shower, chair, floor). Includes functional ambulation and transporting objects" (AOTA, 2014, p. S19).

Moving around in one's environment is essential to taking care of oneself. It is how we move from one self-care activity to another. Think about what you have done thus far today. In your sequence of self-care activities, did they all occur in one place (sitting in the tub) or did you move from place to place and into different positions to accomplish everything? In the field of OT, functional mobility includes not only simply walking, but also moving within occupations. It includes stepping into and out of things, such as a shower or car. It can also include transferring into and out of a wheelchair and moving the chair to do self-care.

Personal Device Care

"Using, cleaning, and maintaining personal care items, such as hearing aids, contact lenses, glasses, orthotics, prosthetics, adaptive equipment, glucometers and contraceptive and sexual devices" (AOTA, 2014, p. S19).

Many people require the use of devices that assist with everyday functioning or compensate for the loss of an ability, such as hearing or vision. In order to stay in working order, these devices must be cared for. For example, eyeglasses become less effective when they are dirty and have smudges across them. Taking a cleaning rag or tissue and cleaning the lenses of eyeglasses would be considered a personal device care activity (Figure 2-3). Earlier, we defined orthotics and prosthetics and how donning and doffing these was considered a dressing activity. Personal device care, such as cleaning and assuring continued functioning of a prosthetic or orthotic device, is recognized as an essential part of self-care.

Personal Hygiene and Grooming

"Obtaining and using supplies; removing body hair (use of razors, tweezers, lotions); applying and removing cosmetics; washing, drying, combing, styling, brushing, and trimming hair; caring for nails (hands and feet); caring for skin, ears, eyes, and nose; applying deodorant; cleaning mouth; brushing and flossing teeth; and removing, cleaning, and reinserting dental orthotics and prosthetics" (AOTA, 2014, p. S19).

The activities required for personal hygiene and grooming are often determined by the individual's gender and culture. The removal of body hair for men may include shaving the face, the chest, or sometimes even the legs and armpits, depending on individual preference. For women, it may include the face (but not as often), eyebrows, legs, and armpits. Removal of this hair can be done in a number of ways, including using a razor (electric or manual), wax, tweezers, or lotions. Applying makeup may or may not be an important activity for women and is done in varying amounts. It is important to notice that hair washing and drying is included in this category and not with bathing/showering. Trimming, filing, and painting the nails is done to preference and is done to both the fingernails and toenails.

Caring for the skin includes not only washing, but also looking for and cleaning any areas that may be at risk for hygiene issues. For example, those with spinal cord injuries must spend time every day inspecting their skin for signs of pressure sores. Many diabetic patients must also spend extra time cleaning and caring for the skin on their feet. Occasionally using a swab, tissue, or other cleaning device to clean the ears and eyes is also essential. Blowing one's nose and removing all mucus is also an activity included in this category. Applying deodorant is often a personal choice and is often culturally guided. Keep in mind that deodorants may be applied in many areas of the body, not just in the axillae. Brushing and care of the teeth is an activity that, in North American cultures, is conducted at least once a day. This includes the cleaning and application of dentures, partial dentures, or dental retainers.

Sexual Activity

"Engaging in activities that result in sexual satisfaction and/or meet relational or reproductive needs" (AOTA, 2014, p. S19).

Sexual satisfaction can be defined in many ways and is unique for each individual. Sexual activity does not have to involve the genitals, nor does it necessarily involve two people. Sexual activity can be part of meeting the needs of a relationship with one or more partners of the same or opposite sex. Sexual activity could also be seen as an activity necessary to meet reproductive needs (i.e., to produce a child). Regardless, the activities surrounding sexual activity are considered part of the ADL, or basic self-care. Thus, sexual activity should be addressed as part of daily life and as a fundamental part of each client's life.

Instrumental Activities of Daily Living

"Activities to support daily life within the home and community that often require more complex interactions than self-care used in ADL" (AOTA, 2014, p. S19).

The IADL are essential to living independently; however, these activities are not necessarily done by the client. For example, many people do not cook their own meals and prefer to eat out or order food for delivery; thus, cooking is not an activity in which they engage. Similarly, car maintenance may be an activity in which many car owners do not engage, instead taking their cars to repair shops for maintenance and repairs. While delegation of many of these activities is an option, overseeing that the activities are completed and delegated to the appropriate people is in itself part of this area of OT.

Care of Others (Including Selecting and Supervising Caregivers)

"Arranging, supervising, or providing the care for others" (AOTA, 2014, p. S19).

This includes caring for an adult family member, spouse, or friend outside of a work setting. The care of another adult can involve providing assistance with any of the previously mentioned self-care activities. It can be as simple as administering medication twice a day or as inclusive as providing total assistance with bathing, toileting, and dressing someone every day. Caregiving is not always conducted long-term but can be done on a temporary basis. This was an occupation that I engaged in for 1 month after my 30-year-old brother had hernia surgery. He needed help cleaning his wound and with meal preparation. Other than that, he was able to handle all of his basic self-care needs. This was an occupation I was not prepared for, yet it was fulfilling and meaningful for me. Note that this category does not include the care of a child; this is explained in the next section.

Child Rearing

"Providing the care and supervision to support the developmental needs of a child" (AOTA, 2014, p. S19).

The *Framework* clarifies that caring for a child goes beyond providing basic self-care needs because it also includes providing adequately for the child's developmental needs (Figure 2-4). Different theorists argue about what contributes to the proper development of a child. However, there are three general parameters to human development: biological, psychological, and social (Hinojosa, Kramer, & Pratt, 1996). Many developmental theories agree that the child must be exposed to appropriate physical and social opportunities to facilitate meeting the developmental milestones typical of a growing child (Hinojosa et al., 1996).

Child rearing also includes supervising and providing care when the primary caregiver is not available. This means finding a preschool or day care facility

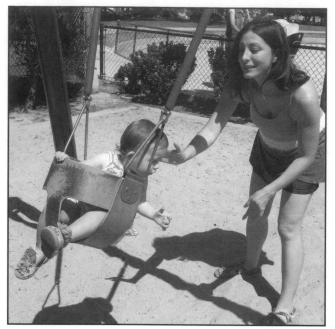

Figure 2-4. Child care includes ensuring proper development through engagement in activities.

while the primary caregiver is away at work or out of the home. Beyond this, it is important to ensure that the alternative caregiver or caregivers meet the developmental needs of the child.

Let's say you have a client, Maura, who has recently been diagnosed with depression. She has an 18-month-old daughter named Bethie who lives with her in her apartment. Maura gives Bethie her bottle every 3 hours. She has not yet started her on solid foods. Bethie spends most of her day strapped into a high chair because Maura is afraid that Bethie will hurt herself if she allowed to be on the ground. Maura spends all day watching TV and has not been out of the house in weeks. What is Maura doing to support the developmental needs of her child? Is this an area of occupation Maura is having difficulty with?

Care of Pets

"Arranging, supervising, or providing the care for pets and service animals" (AOTA, 2014, p. S19).

The task required of providing care for a pet is different for each person. There are factors that may vary the amount and types of tasks, but generally most animals require at the very least food, water, safe shelter, and care of health needs. There may be many other tasks required, depending on the animal, the environment it lives in, and its particular demands.

For example, a horse requires a greater amount of care than perhaps a cat does (except for especially spoiled and demanding cats). Just as with the child-rearing category, this includes finding and supervising the care of these pets if the primary owner is not able. So while I am on vacation, I must arrange for someone competent and reliable to come to my home to feed and water my cats and clean the litter box. (Finding someone to play with them for a while also assures that my sofa will not be ripped to shreds when I return.)

Communication Management

"Sending, receiving and interpreting information using a variety of systems and equipment including writing tools, telephones (cell phones/ smart phones), keyboards, audiovisual recorders, computers/tablets, communication boards, call lights, emergency systems, Braille writers, telecommunication devices for the deaf, augmentative communication systems, and personal digital assistants" (AOTA, 2014, p. S19).

Multiple devices are used to relay information from one person to another. Over the last few decades, technological advances have given us greater and faster ways to communicate with others. Technology has begun to advance so quickly that new ways of communicating may have been developed by the time this book has been printed and reached your hands. Humans communicate using cellular, wireless, or standard (i.e., landline) phones and using the Internet via computers, tablets, phones, or other devices. Typewriters are still occasionally used, as well as word processors to print out text. Call lights or emergency systems are used by those who are in bed, on a commode, or unable to move from a given location to notify others that they need assistance. These are used not only in hospitals and medical settings, but also within homes. These call lights or emergency systems are often activated by pulling a cord or pushing a button, which in turn creates a noise or flashing light to signal others that help is needed.

Alternative communication devices are used by those who are unable to speak or hear. Communication boards are simple one-dimensional pieces of paper or boards with the alphabet or common words or objects printed on them. The user will point to or indicate which object or letter he or she is trying to convey to another person. Higher-tech options are available that have voice output, speaking a word or words aloud. These devices can be activated via a number of user abilities, including movement, breath, or noise. Communication devices for those who are hard of hearing or deaf include adaptive telephones that allow the user to receive communication via typed-in text from an operator and to respond through either speech or typing. For more information regarding these devices and the area of assistive technology, please refer to *Assistive Technologies: Principles and Practice* (Cook & Polgar, 2008).

Driving and Community Mobility

"Planning and moving around in the community and using public or private transportation, such as driving, walking, bicycling, or accessing and riding buses, taxi cabs, or other public transportation systems" (AOTA, 2014, p. S19).

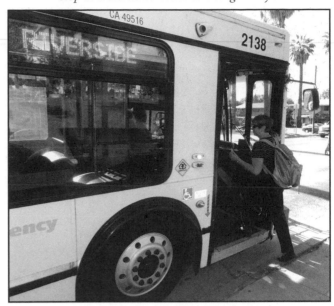

Figure 2-5. Getting on a bus as community mobility.

While mobility was discussed in the category of ADL, it was on a more personal basis. Community mobility involves the person outside of the home and in areas of the person's community. Getting to and from places such as church, school, or the grocery store is essential to many people's lives. However, driving independently is not always an option. Using a bus, taxicab, subway, or transportation service for the disabled are other options to allow a person to engage in this occupation (Figure 2-5). The use of each of these methods requires different tasks. For example, to use a public bus, a person must first find a schedule indicating which bus and route will take him or her to the desired destination. He or she must get to the bus stop at the appropriate time, have the correct fare for the round trip, and be able to get onto the bus. He or she must pay the bus driver for the ride and be able to recognize when to get off the bus.

Financial Management

"Using fiscal resources, including alternate methods of financial transaction and planning and using finances with long-term and short-term goals" (AOTA, 2014, p. S19).

Taking care of personal finances is now conducted in many different ways. In the past, bills were paid using a checkbook, stamps, and envelopes. Now, many people use online bill-paying services that are run through banks. This eliminates the need to write out checks and stuff and stamp envelopes. For those with physical disabilities, it has made bill paying much easier. However, financial management goes beyond just paying bills and includes making sure that the money available will meet current needs, as well as

help to meet future needs and goals. Thus, planning and saving for the future; managing investments, alternative income, or savings; and filing income tax are also considered tasks.

Health Management and Maintenance

"Developing, managing, and maintaining routines for health and wellness promotion, such as physical fitness, nutrition, decreasing health risk behaviors, and medication routines" (AOTA, 2014, p. S19).

The level at which one manages and maintains his or her health varies from person to person. Some see this as a priority and spend great amounts of time exercising and eating well. Examples of activities considered part of health management and maintenance include observing and conducting any medical needs (such as a person with diabetes checking blood sugar levels and administering insulin), taking vitamins or medications, and applying topical medications.

Home Establishment and Management

"Obtaining and maintaining personal and household possessions and environment (e.g., home, yard, garden, appliances, vehicles), including maintaining and repairing personal possessions (e.g., clothing, household items) and knowing how to seek help or whom to contact" (AOTA, 2014, p. S19).

ACTIVITY 2-3

Suzanna is an 18-year-old who is 6 months pregnant. When her parents found out she was pregnant, they kicked her out of their home, and she is now in a homeless shelter. What tasks does Suzanna have ahead of her in order to obtain housing for her and her future child?

_____

_____

_____

_____

_____

_____

_____

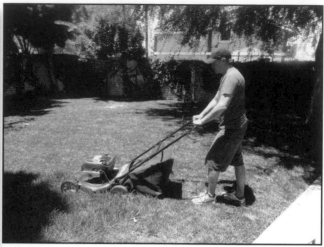

Figure 2-6. Mowing the lawn.

Finding a place to live and keeping it safe to live in is an occupation that many young adults adopt as they mature and decide to live on their own (Activity 2-3). This occupation encompasses three major areas: (1) finding and obtaining a place to live, (2) maintaining the household environment, and (3) maintaining and repairing objects that are personal possessions. How a person defines home will define the activities required of finding a home. The activities required of a student moving out of his or her parents' home for the first time are much different than those of an elderly person who is no longer safe staying in his or her home of 40 years and must move into a nursing home.

Once a person has established a place of residence, varying amounts of maintenance are required to keep the environment safe and up to required standards, dependent on the community. For example, some neighborhoods have requirements for lawn and exterior home upkeep, meaning the lawn must be mowed (Figure 2-6), weeds pulled, and the paint on the house kept up. For many, this upkeep is not forced by regulations but is viewed as part of the role of homeowner (or even renter). The actual tasks of maintaining the exterior home environment (mowing the lawn, pulling weeds, etc.) do not necessarily need to be done by the person but are arranged to be completed by someone else. Thus, part of this area of occupation is finding

help for these tasks (e.g., calling a gardener or hiring the teenager next door to mow the lawn).

Maintenance of a home also includes ensuring that the interior is kept in repair and safe. Thus, cleaning, mopping, vacuuming, dusting, and picking up trash are a few of the activities included as part of this area of occupation. While people engage in this occupation to varying degrees (and enjoy it in even greater degrees of variation), it is still essential to living in a healthy environment. Also, part of this area of occupation is the concept of maintaining or repairing possessions. This can include clothing (laundering and storing), automobiles, appliances, and all objects within the home.

For all of the activities in this area of occupation, the person does not have to do the actual maintenance or repair but simply must know when and how to address it and obtain assistance when needed. Even in a small studio apartment, one needs to know what to do when a light bulb burns out or the hot water stops working.

A person's ability to maintain his or her home environment is often one of the first occupations to deteriorate with the onset of an illness or the progression of a disease. Limitations can be caused not only by physical limitations, but also by cognitive or mental health issues. For example, Nancy and Bob have been married for 56 years. Both have shared the activities encompassing home maintenance, with each taking responsibility for different aspects. While Bob made sure that the yard was always well groomed, the peach trees were trimmed, the snow was shoveled from the driveway, and the appliances were in working order, Nancy took care of the interior of the home, doing the family laundry and keeping the bathrooms and living areas clean. Nancy was diagnosed with Alzheimer's disease 4 years earlier. As the disease progressed, Bob found that Nancy was leaving many of the cleaning tasks uncompleted or undone. Dust began to build on the bookshelves, and dog hair began to build up so thick on the couch that it looked a different color. Bob walked into the basement one day to find the floor covered with soap bubbles. Mary had mistakenly put dish soap into the clothes washing machine. Although Nancy had completed these occupations for so many years, Bob decided to have a housekeeper come once a week to help complete some of the activities Nancy was struggling with. Bob made sure that his home was properly maintained and cared for by recognizing what was needed in order to be safe and contacting someone for assistance.

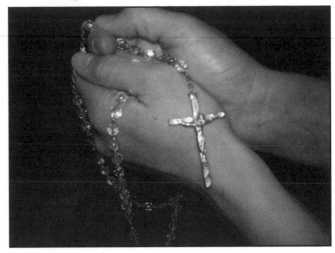

Figure 2-7. Praying the rosary.

Meal Preparation and Cleanup

"Planning, preparing, serving well-balanced, nutritional meals and cleaning up food and utensils after meals" (AOTA, 2014, p. S20).

Much like home maintenance and repair, meal preparation is done in varying degrees by different people. Meal preparation begins with the process of deciding what to prepare and what items and ingredients are needed. Interestingly, this area of occupation is defined as concerning only "well-balanced, nutritional meals." For many (especially busy students), meal preparation entails obtaining nourishment in forms that would not be considered well balanced. Nonetheless, meal preparation, or cooking, is done in a variety of ways. Meal preparation includes not only the preparation of food, but also serving it in the appropriate dish, bowl, or platter. For example, the making and serving of soup is only complete when it is poured into bowls. After a meal is eaten, all materials and objects that were used in the process must be cleaned up. This includes washing all dishes and utensils, putting away any unused food, and wiping up the surfaces that were used. While some of the tasks included here sound much like the cleaning tasks included under "home management," because they may occur during the process of preparing a meal or are done in conjunction with the completion, they are considered part of this occupation. Not included in this occupation is the activity of eating and feeding. The process of creating food for consumption does not include the person eating it. You may encounter clients who enjoy the occupation of meal preparation but not eating, or vice versa.

Religious and Spiritual Activities and Expression

"Participating in religion, an organized system of beliefs, practices, rituals, and symbols designed to facilitate closeness to the sacred or transcendent (Moreira-Almeida & Koenig, 2006, p. 844) and engaging in activities that allow a sense of connectedness to something larger than oneself or that are especially meaningful, such as taking time out to play with a child, engaging in activities in nature, and helping others in need (Spencer, Davidson, & White, 1997)" (AOTA, 2014, p. S20).

Religious occupations are those activities surrounding involvement in organized rituals or practices that are used to demonstrate beliefs (Billock, 2009). It is often through the religious occupations that many hope to reach a greater understanding of the spiritual self and gain a sense of something greater than themselves.

There are thousands of organized religions, each with their own set of rituals and practices. For some, there are weekly meetings or church services. It is during these meetings that there are actions and behaviors expected of those attending. In some church services, there is singing, reading, listening to a sermon, and reading verses or incantations aloud. Physical actions such as kneeling or moving through a series of motions a certain number of times can be required. A very common physical activity for Catholics is holding a rosary, which is a cross on a string of 59 beads (Figure 2-7). The string of beads is held and manipulated as a prayer is said for each bead. Other religious activities include attending classes, going to confession, praying, and reading the Bible or other materials. There are also some religions that utilize animal sacrifice as part of their rituals.

Religion is used as a way to reach into the spiritual aspects of the self; however, spiritual experiences do not necessarily need to occur during religious occupations (Billock, 2014). The terms *spirituality* and *religion* are often misinterpreted as meaning the same thing. While they are related, spirituality is an internal experience, a "personal quest for understanding answers to ultimate questions about life, about meaning, and the sacred" (Moyers & Dale, 2007, p. 28). Spirituality is not an activity or occupation but rather occurs within the person as a result of engagement in occupations. We experience meaning by engaging in occupations that take us away from ourselves, make us lose our sense of time, or give us a sense of connectedness with others. This inner experience that occurs during meaningful occupations is often what brings us back to engaging in these occupations throughout our lives. It is the occupations that take our breath away, bring us to tears, or simply answer ultimate questions about life that have spiritual meaning, whether we recognize it or not. Those activities that are spiritual in nature will often reveal themselves during the occupational profile. For example, 22-year-old David tells his OT that he really enjoys going to dance clubs and dancing. When asked why, he states, "I like feeling like one with the crowd. The energy of the music and the people takes me to another place." For David, dancing at dance clubs is a spiritual experience, though not one that we might instinctually think of a spiritual.

Consider times in your life when you were engaged in an activity and found yourself emotionally moved. Think back to the times when you were happiest and most fulfilled; what were you doing? Perhaps you did not consider these spiritual moments, but in the context of occupational fulfillment, these were spiritual experiences. For our clients, not being able to engage in activities that bring their lives meaning leaves them with a huge loss in that they are less able to find meaning in life.

Safety and Emergency Maintenance

"Knowing and performing preventive procedures to maintain a safe environment; recognizing sudden, unexpected hazardous situations and initiating emergency action to reduce the threat to health and safety; examples include ensuring safety when entering and exiting the

home, identifying emergency contact numbers, and replacing items such as batteries in smoke alarms and light bulbs" (AOTA, 2014, p. S20).

The activities that comprise this type of occupation are either ongoing preventative measures or immediate reactions to emergency situations. Ongoing preventative measures are taken to ensure that the environments the person is in are safe from immediate or eventual danger. It requires that the person understand threats to safety and how to prevent them. For example, a person must know that he or she must not set newspaper on top of a stove. Safety procedures are often incorporated within other occupations, such as meal preparation.

Shopping

"Preparing shopping lists (grocery and other); selecting, purchasing and transporting items; selecting method of payment; and completing money transactions; included are Internet shopping and related use of electronic devices such as computers, cellular telephones, and tablets" (AOTA, 2014, p. S20).

Purchasing items or services is often what provides the items needed for survival, such as food, water, and clothing. It is also a form of leisure and enjoyment for many people, when items are purchased for other reasons other than for survival. For example, Carey wants to purchase a new video game. This is not necessary for Carey's survival (although he may try to convince his wife otherwise). In order to purchase the game, he will need to find a place where it is sold. There are multiple ways in which shopping can occur: in a store, online, from a catalog, from a salesperson, via the phone, from a personal ad (either placed in a newspaper or online), from a yard sale, or at an outdoor market. Let's say Carey decides to purchase the video game online. He would need to look at the prices from different vendors to find the lowest price. He would need to choose a method of payment, which is usually via credit card when purchasing online. Completing the purchase would require providing the appropriate credit card and shipping information. If Carey was not able to purchase the game online, he might chose to go to a store. If so, he would need to navigate within the store in order to find the game he is looking for. He would take the game to a checkout counter and pay the attendant with cash, credit, or a check. However, having an attendant at the checkout counter is optional at some stores, as self-checkout machines are becoming more common in larger department stores. This would require Carey to scan in the game and follow the directions on a screen to provide payment.

Rest and Sleep

"Activities related to obtaining restorative rest and sleep that supports healthy, active engagement in other occupations" (AOTA, 2014, p. S20).

Rest

"Engaging in quiet and effortless actions that interrupt physical and mental activity resulting in a relaxed state (Nurit & Michel, 2003, p. 227); included are identifying the need to relax; reducing involvement in taxing physical, mental, or social activities; and engaging in relaxation or other endeavors that restore energy, calm, and renewed interest in engagement" (AOTA, 2014, p. S20).

Humans require periods of inactivity within their day in order to function (Figure 2-8). By resting, we allow our bodies to regain energy to reengage in activities. Physical and mental activity can be taxing over a period of time. The amount of rest required is often greater for some people than others, such as with those recovering from an illness and with decreased physical, cognitive, or aerobic capacity. Physical rest occurs by allowing muscle tension to reduce and the number of muscle contractions to decrease. For example, if one is standing for long periods, a rest may include sitting or lying down. Mental rest occurs by allowing little to no mental processing of information or problem solving. People choose to engage in this occupation in many ways. For many Americans, watching television is the favored way to rest. Watching television allows for passive engagement in an activity that utilizes only sensory processing of what is seen and heard. The body is allowed to be inactive while cognitive abilities are minimally challenged. For some, television is not considered restful or relaxing. For those people, greater quiet and relaxation are required in order to fully allow the mind and body to rest. Meditation and visual imagery are examples of activities some people use to engage in rest (this may also be considered a spiritual occupation for some).

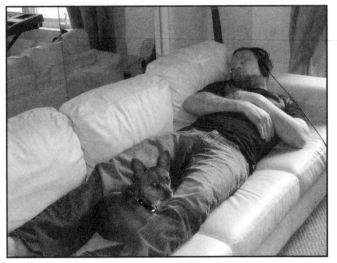

Figure 2-8. Resting.

Sleep Preparation: Defined in Two Parts

"(1) Engaging in routines that prepare the self for a comfortable rest, such as grooming and undressing, reading or listening to music to fall asleep, saying goodnight to others, engaging in meditation or prayers; determining the time of day and length of time desired for sleeping or the time needed to wake; and establishing sleep patterns that support growth and health (patterns are often personally and culturally determined)" (AOTA, 2014, p. S20).

The activities leading up to engagement in sleep have been divided into two separate categories. The first category is related to preparing the body and mind for the occupation of sleep, and the second is related to preparing the environment. Preparing the body includes activities such as removing clothes worn during the rest of the day and donning sleepwear, brushing teeth, and washing the face or body. These activities are performed in order to facilitate a more restful experience. For example, changing out of the clothes that were worn all day allows the body to be relieved of any uncomfortable sensory input and thus allows for a deeper and more comfortable sleep. Many of these activities become part of a daily pattern and are routine, with the same activities occurring every day prior to going to sleep.

The mind is prepared for sleep by engaging in relaxing activities that allow thought patterns to slow down and retreat. The slowing of our thought processes occurs as we relax and approach a state of sleep. How one reaches this relaxed state varies according to

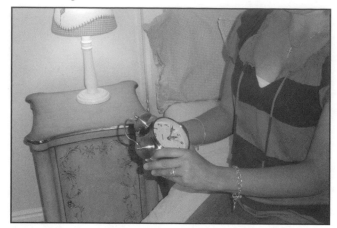

Figure 2-9. Setting the alarm clock to prepare for sleep.

personal beliefs and values. It is also dependent upon how well one is able to calm the mind to the point of giving up consciousness. Some people require a time of quiet activity, such as reading or listening to music, before retiring to sleep. Another technique often utilized to this effect is meditation or visualization.

Consciously deciding to go to sleep is also part of the mental processes required for sleep preparation. Choosing when to sleep and wake allows for the establishment of sleep/wake cycles that are healthy and provide adequate opportunity for the body to rejuvenate. This occurs with an average of 6 to 8 hours of continuous sleep. For this to take place, one must plan the time during the 24-hour period that will allow for this (Figure 2-9). If a person must be awake at 7 a.m., he or she must prepare to be asleep by 11 p.m. in order to get 8 hours of sleep. Mentally processing this is an activity that is part of the preparations for healthy sleep. For people with the inability to schedule 6 to 8 hours of sleep, scheduling sleep may be more difficult. This is the case for those who work in jobs that demand long shifts and scattered windows of time in which to sleep. Crab fishermen often work 24- to 30-hour shifts with little to no sleep and must schedule intermittent nap periods while their boats travel from one fishing spot to another.

> *"(2) Preparing the physical environment for periods of unconsciousness, such as making the bed or space on which to sleep; ensuring warmth/coolness and protection; setting an alarm clock; securing the home, such as locking doors or closing windows or curtains; and turning off electronics or lights"* (AOTA, 2014, p. S20).

By ensuring a comfortable and secure environment, one facilitates the ability to engage in sleep and stay asleep. This requires reducing the amount of sensory stimuli during the time in which sleep occurs. Limiting the amount of light in the area may require closing window blinds or doors and shutting off lights. Removing other arousing stimuli from the environment (or removing the person from the stimulating environment) will also allow for a greater ability to engage in sleep. For example, for a person trying to sleep, a crying puppy would be a distraction from full engagement in sleep. Other aspects of the environment—such as thermal regulation or modifying how much the body will be exposed to heat or cold during sleep—involve adjusting and setting any environmental heating or cooling equipment as well as providing an appropriate covering for the body during sleep. Most important of all of the physical preparations is finding a place to lay the body, such as on a bed or other surface. For most people, this means pulling back the covers and sheets on a bed to open up enough space in which to lie down and then pulling the covers back up and over the body.

Sleep Participation

> *"Taking care of personal need for sleep such as ceasing activities to ensure onset of sleep, napping, dreaming; sustaining a sleep state without disruption; and performing nighttime care of toileting needs and hydration; also negotiating the needs and requirement of and interacting with others within the social environment such as children or partners, including providing nighttime caregiving such as breastfeeding and monitoring the comfort and safety of others who are sleeping"* (AOTA, 2014, p. S20).

Since its genesis as a profession, OT has espoused the importance of a balance of work, rest, and play. However, it was not until the second edition of the *Framework* that sleep was identified as an occupation and thus part of OT's domain. Sleep science studies have identified the value that sleep has for physical and mental health (McKnight-Eily et al., 2008). Although it is an occupation that is essential to well-being, the role of OT with regard to sleep is just beginning to emerge (West, 2009).

While engaged in sleep, the body and mind are at rest, with the eyes closed, and there is little or no response to the external environment. It is during sleep that the brain develops unique cycles of brain wave activity, with periods of dreaming. It is disengagement from the external environment that begins the process of allowing the mind and body to be at rest. To allow the mind to become unconscious, one must allow the brain to release control over staying alert to internal and external stimuli (*Mosby's Dictionary*, 2006). Engagement in a sleep state might be impaired by internal stimuli such as pain, in which the brain continues to process information from the body. In order for this occupation to be successful, both the body and mind must disengage from activity.

The actual participation in sleep includes ensuring that there is adequate engagement in the activity and allowing for necessary actions while sleeping. While engaging in sleep, we move, interact with others, and respond appropriately to external stimuli as needed. For example, once we are immersed in sleep, we unconsciously regulate our activities and responses to ensure the continuation of sleep cycles. For example, we may turn our bodies in our sleep when we sense discomfort. We may put an arm or leg around the person sleeping next to us or even pull up the covers without ever becoming fully conscious. We may disrupt sleep to get up and use the bathroom. Upon certain sounds or sensations (such as hearing a baby cry or an alarm go off), we alert ourselves to action to become fully alert.

Education

> *"Activities needed for learning and participating in the educational environment"* (AOTA, 2014, p. S20).

Formal Educational Participation

> *"Participating in academic (e.g., math, reading, degree coursework), nonacademic (e.g., recess, lunchroom, hallway), extracurricular (e.g., sports, band, cheerleading, dances), and vocational (prevocational and vocational) educational activities"* (AOTA, 2014, p. S20).

The activities that encompass attending an educational program or school include not only the academic aspects of learning and participation, but also the out-of-classroom activities such as recess and mealtimes. Activities that may occur outside of class time—such as being part of a school band, being on a school sports team, and attending school functions such as a dance or other social event—are all part of being a student. It is through all of these activities that students learn about the world and how to interact with those around them. Some educational programs provide training for certain jobs or professions and may include on-the-job training or internships.

Samantha is 5 years old and just started kindergarten. She found that the activities that occur during kindergarten are much different than what was happening at home. She starts her day by getting on the school bus that picks her up at the end of her block. She must patiently wait for the bus and board in an orderly fashion. She must find a seat and sit in the seat while the bus transports her to school, making a few stops on the way to pick up other students. When at school, she must find her classroom and put her backpack at her desk. She must listen for when the bell rings, which means that it is time for class to start. She participates in many activities during class time, learning how to write letters and how to share with others. When she needs to use the restroom, she must ask the teacher for permission. She takes herself to the bathroom and comes back to the classroom when finished. At snack time, she goes to the cafeteria, where she must pick up a container of milk or juice and one cracker. During recess, she plays with other children, learning how to interact and share equipment and toys. When the day is over, she gets back on the bus and must exit the bus at the same point she got on, at the end of her block. All of these activities are part of her participation in formal education (Activity 2-4).

Informal Personal Educational Needs or Exploration of Interests (Beyond Formal Education)

> *"Identifying topics and methods for obtaining topic-related information or skills"* (AOTA, 2014, p. S20).

Education outside of a formal setting occurs in many different venues and ways. If knowledge is needed in a particular area, the specific topics must be identified in order to determine methods whereby it may be acquired. For example, Jean is an occupational therapist who has decided that she would like to travel to Haiti to work as a volunteer. In order to fully understand what she needs to know before she goes, she contacts another occupational therapist who has already traveled and worked there. She finds that she needs to be prepared to speak basic Haitian Creole, the native

ACTIVITY 2-4

List all of the activities or tasks that are required for your engagement in formal educational participation right now:

_____

_____

_____

_____

_____

_____

language. Jean does an Internet search for Haitian Creole lessons and finds a podcast series to download. All of these activities were in preparation for the informal education she hopes to engage in. Exploring the different methods whereby to gain information is much more extensive and yet much easier in many ways now that so much information is posted on the Internet. An Internet search can provide information on a wide variety of topics, what the prerequisites are to pursue a specific topic, and where to gain further information. A search on one topic may lead to ideas for other topics. Searching the Internet is only one way of exploring informal education. Talking to others, calling organizations, and reading the newspaper are all examples of how informal education topics can be researched and discovered.

Informal Personal Education Participation

"Participating in informal classes, programs, and activities that provide instruction or training in identified areas of interest" (AOTA, 2014, p. S20).

The ways in which we are able to engage in learning have evolved over the years, enabling us to acquire knowledge almost anywhere. For example, Jean wanted to learn basic Creole. She managed to do so by listening to the lessons on her MP3 player while on her hour-long commute each day. Informal education

occurs in classrooms and homes, on street corners, and at senior centers, just to name a few. Learning any new thing can occur independently of others by engaging in activities that encourage learning, such as reading, listening to audiotapes, or learning through engagement in the activity and improving one's skill by trial and error. Participation in informal education can occur in conjunction with or guided by others. Classes or instruction may be led by a teacher or guided by students with greater experience.

Informal education includes gaining a skill or knowledge that is not part of a formal educational program. Interests outside of formal educational can include leisure, social, or health-related topics. Classes in yoga, kickboxing, painting, and English as a second language are all examples of informal education. Informal education includes not only the classes, but also the activities that facilitate the learning process. For example, Jill, who is 38 years old, has always wanted to learn how to play the piano. She began taking weekly piano lessons from a neighbor. Her engagement in this learning was not limited to those weekly lessons but also included daily practice on her piano. After 6 months of lessons, she performed at her first recital, having learned to play one of her daughter's favorite songs (Activity 2-5).

Work

"Labor or exertion; to make, construct, manufacture, form, fashion or shape objects; to organize, plan, or evaluate services or processes of living or governing; committed occupations that are performed with or without financial reward (Christiansen & Townsend, 2010, p. 423)" (AOTA, 2014, p. S20).

Employment Interests and Pursuits

"Identifying and selecting work opportunities based on personal assets, limitations, likes, and dislikes relative to work (adapted from Mosey, 1996, p. 342)" (AOTA, 2014, p. S20).

How did you decide to become an occupational therapist or OTA? Did you look for jobs that addressed your strengths and weaknesses? Did you talk to others who are in the field? Perhaps you found out about OT through personal experience. Once you decided that this was the profession you wanted to get into, how did you find about the requirements for practice? The identification of work options involves finding work or career opportunities that match the individual's personality traits and desires. Finding out about a career can occur spontaneously or by chance, as when listening to the radio, watching TV, or encountering the profession through life experiences. The exploration of career options can also occur through deliberate investigation by taking competency and job matching assessments. Some people go through job counseling with a career counselor to find the right match.

Employment Seeking and Acquisition

"Advocating for oneself; completing, submitting, and reviewing appropriate application materials, preparing for interviews, participating in interviews; participating in interviews and following up afterward; discussing job benefits, and finalizing negotiations" (AOTA, 2014, p. S20).

Once an area of work is identified, pursuing that career or job requires searching and identifying job opportunities that are available. This is done in many ways, including searching the Internet, reading the newspaper, looking at job postings, and talking to human resources or recruiting departments. Pursuing a particular job may require personally speaking to someone from companies that the person wishes to work for, as not all job opportunities are posted or readily available to the public.

Obtaining employment once a job opportunity has been identified involves a number of common activities that are required for most jobs. Of course, each job opening may have different requirements of the applicant, so the first step to seeking out employment for a particular opening would be to ascertain what is required to apply for the job. Most employers require an employment application to be completed, either with pen and paper or on the Internet. The application must be submitted to the appropriate department or employee. Along with the application, some employers require other materials to be submitted, such as a résumé, background check, or sample work. After the application is accepted, the next step may be an interview, which can occur in person, over the phone, or via the Internet. The applicant prepares for this interview by gathering information regarding the company and job position and by thinking about how he or she might answer questions during the interview. The appropriate clothing must be selected for the interview

---

ACTIVITY 2-5

List informal classes or workshops that you have attended that would be considered informal education participation:

_____

_____

_____

_____

_____

_____

---

if it will occur in person or via a webcam. For some job openings, a series of interviews may be held, with some of these comprising a group, where multiple applicants are interviewed at the same time. Testing or competency assessments that precede or follow the interview are part of some job application processes.

Job Performance

"Performing the requirements of a job, including work skills and patterns, time management; relationships with co-workers, managers, and customers; leadership and supervision; creation, production, and distribution of products and services; initiation, sustainment, and completion of work; and compliance with work norms and procedures" (AOTA, 2014, p. S20).

Once employment is obtained, remaining employed requires that the employee meet the expectations of the employer. This means that the employee must maintain regular work habits, including punctuality (coming to work and leaving on time) and being productive in the assigned job while at work. For each job, these expectations will be different, according to the type of work, the setting, and the employer's expectations. There are some employers who do not expect employees to arrive at a certain time every day but have high expectations of their employees' productivity once

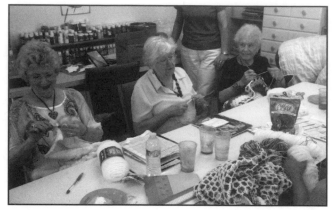

Figure 2-10. A group of retired women enjoying engaging in a knitting group.

they are at work. These employers believe in quality and quantity of work, not the number of hours it takes to get the work done. However, this does not work in every setting, and for most western jobs, specific hours are determined for employees. Job performance may require engaging in activities involving a variety of skills, including motor movements, cognitive processing, and social interaction. Social interaction may occur between the employee and customers, with others in the community, or with other employees (not to mention the employer and supervisors). The expectation for social interaction varies according to the degree to which the employee is required to interact with others, as well as the culture of the environment. In some settings, the use of foul language and yelling may be acceptable, while in others this sort of thing would be grounds for termination. The activities and level of skill needed depend on the type of job and the expectations of the employer. The employee must understand these expectations and meet them in order to maintain his or her employment.

Retirement Preparation and Adjustment

"Determining aptitudes, developing interest and skills, and selecting appropriate avocational pursuits, and adjusting lifestyle in the absence of the worker role" (AOTA, 2014, p. S20).

Retirement is the voluntary discontinuation of employment, or complete cessation of work, that typically occurs at age 65 years or older. For many people, work provides a sense of efficacy, an avenue for socialization, and self-esteem (McMinn, 2009). Without activities to replace these needs, many retired people decline in physical and mental health (Dave,

Rashad, & Spasojevic, 2008). Depression is very common among those who retire; often they do not find adequate ways in which to fill the needs that were met through work.

Filling the void that is left by retirement can be done in many ways. This time, which is no longer dedicated to work, is seen by many as a time to engage in those activities that they did not have time for while working full time, such as traveling, participating in leisure activities, or volunteering for philanthropic organizations or causes. Healthy transition from the role of worker to retiree requires preplanning—setting future goals and desires for those occupations and roles that will meet intrinsic needs. Socioeconomic status plays a large part in these plans, as income stream shifts from receiving a paycheck to social security payments and any retirement funds the person had set aside. Many retirees have difficulty meeting expenses with the extreme cut in income, with some entering into poverty. Physical health may limit retirement adjustment if mobility, pain, or physical weaknesses restrict the ability to engage in desired occupations.

Community resources and access to environments that lend themselves to productive retirement also influence adjustment to this role shift. For those in rural areas, there is limited access to community activities, and public transportation outside of the home may be restricted. However, even without access to community, activities around the home can fill the day with meaning. For example, Mildred was a full-time elementary school teacher in a small farm town. She and her husband live on 500 acres of farm land 20 miles from town. Now that she and her husband are retired, they love to go fishing at the local lake, camping in their RV, and spending time with their grandchildren. Mildred has a garden that requires constant attention during the spring and summer months; she is always also making a quilt or blanket (Figure 2-10) and has started her own line of underwear and tops, which she sells at the local market. Mildred states, "I am busier now than when I was working."

Mildred is at one end of the spectrum of retirement adjustment, while at the other lie those who do little with the time they now have. These are people who had little planned for retirement or have little desire to engage in anything other than rest. Ernie is Mildred's former employer who lives a few miles down the road. At Ernie's retirement party, he told Mildred, "All I am going to do when I retire is sit and rock in my rocking chair." For 3 years now, that is what Ernie has done every day; he sits in his rocking chair and watches television. Ernie's plan for transition from the role of principal of an elementary school to retiree did not include replacing the intrinsic rewards he gained from work; it was a choice he made without realizing the difficulties he might encounter in adjusting to this new role. Common to many retirees, adjusting to the absence of the worker role can cause a decline in physical and mental health.

Planning for retirement requires looking for new roles and occupations that provide enriching experiences to help support health. This includes matching one's strengths and abilities to opportunities that align with one's interests. Retirement can also be a time in which skills can be gained or knowledge sought. An assessment of life goals, what a person hopes to have accomplished in life, can lead to finding those meaningful occupations to pursue during the retirement years. Re-exploring past occupations and interests, such as those engaged in earlier in life, is often part of successful retirement planning. OT practitioners address these occupations with clients who may be entering into this stage of life by using assessments that evaluate interests and abilities and matching these up to possible occupations. Constructing a "productive day" schedule, which gives the retiree a routine and tasks to do throughout the week, can be created with the client. These are just a few examples of how OT plays a role in retirement planning and they also show how a person can engage in a new occupation on his or her own to ensure healthy adjustment to retirement.

Volunteer Exploration

"Determining community causes, organizations, or opportunities for unpaid work in relationship to personal skills, interest, location, and time available" (AOTA, 2014, p. S21).

Prior to engagement in volunteerism, the potential volunteer must explore the different types of philanthropic work available and determine what he or she deems as worth contributing time to. Volunteer work is often done in efforts to increase the well-being of humanity or improve conditions in what one believes to be an issue or charity in need. Skills offered by volunteers range from stuffing envelopes and making phone calls to being a board member of a nonprofit hospital or serving as a physician in a Third World country. Finding opportunities for volunteerism can occur through active or passive mechanisms. Active

pursuit of volunteer opportunities occurs when the potential volunteer seeks out volunteer organizations and opportunities based on his or her skill set and the time he or she is willing to contribute. For example, a person may decide that he or she wants to work with underprivileged or at-risk youth and therefore contacts the local high school or Boys and Girls Club. Volunteer opportunities also present themselves in the communities or organizations in which potential volunteers already participate. For example, a mother may be asked to serve in her daughter's Girl Scout troop. As a passively presented volunteer opportunity, the mother would then explore this volunteer opportunity to determine if it would be a good fit with her skills and available time.

Volunteer Participation

"Performing unpaid work activities for the benefit of selected causes, organizations, or facilities" (AOTA, 2014, p. S21).

Once a volunteer opportunity has been explored and identified, participation entails much of what a paid work position might. Volunteer positions have varying expectations of participation; the level at which this occurs varies according to the role the volunteer plays and the organization. A volunteer who leads a weekly community yoga class will have different expectations from those of the president of the AOTA (also a volunteer position!). The demands for those activities involved should match the volunteer's abilities and time available (as was addressed in the precursor to this occupation—volunteer exploration).

Play

"Any spontaneous or organized activity that provides enjoyment, entertainment, amusement, or diversion (Parham & Fazio, 1997, p. 252)" (AOTA, 2014, p. S21).

What defines play and how it is different from leisure has been a debate evident in the literature for years. Definitions of play range from focusing on the activities of children to spontaneous action that provides enjoyment. However, in observing a group of adults playing laser tag, one can assert that no one definition seems appropriate. At what point in human development do we stop playing and start engaging in leisure? While play is the primary occupation of children, it is an occupation that can be engaged in across the life span.

Play and its impact on humans has been an area of study for many scientists, who have identified some key elements of play that correspond and are agreed upon by most theories and definitions of play. Play activities are engaged in for intrinsic rewards, such as happiness or excitement, not for external rewards or gains. Play is also focused on the process or the "doing" of the activity versus an end result. Play activities are also those that are freely chosen rather than engaged in because of expectations or requirements. The most essential characteristic of play is that it provides enjoyment or pleasure (Parham, 2008). While other occupations may provoke these emotions, play is not possible without enjoyment or pleasure and is the primary motivator toward engagement in play. For example, we may feel enjoyment or pleasure while cooking or working, but it is not our primary motivation in engaging in it. For some people, cooking can have many aspects of play, but it is a leisure activity or an IADL because the focus is on the end result. We further define the characteristics of leisure later in this chapter.

Play Exploration

"Identifying appropriate play activities, which can include exploration play, practice play, pretend play, games with rules, constructive play, and symbolic play (adapted from Bergen, 1988, pp. 64-65)" (AOTA, 2014, p. S21).

To thoroughly understand the scope and breadth of the complexity of play, one could read hundreds of books and journals on the topic. The *Framework* introduces us to some of the basic concepts of play and the different forms that the occupation of play can take. Play exploration is differentiated as an occupation separate from participation in play in that play exploration activities are the child's or adult's actions toward investigating and choosing play activities. A child may begin one play activity and then shift to another based on intrinsic needs or developmental level. When an individual is involved in social play (play conducted with others), play exploration requires collaborating with other children or adults to determine the play activities.

The *Framework* presents six different types of play that have been named and defined by different theories. Jean Piaget, a developmental psychologist, fathered foundational theories that emphasized that cognitive development occurred out of play experiences. Over the years, other theorists have utilized Piaget's play theory as a basis for development of other theories, which include fundamental aspects of how the play experience contributes to human development. Out of these theories, several categories or types of play have been identified, which change as a child develops and ages (Knox, 2005).

Practice play, which typically occurs from infancy to age 2 years, includes activities that are conducted for the sake of experiencing the effect. This is often termed *sensorimotor play*, as this type of play includes exploring sensations and how the body moves (Parham, 2008). Mary Reilly termed this type of play *exploratory play*, which she believed to encompass more than cognitive development and is a means by which a child seeks to understand his or her environment and sensory experiences (Parham, 2008). This type of play behavior is strictly intrinsically motivated, as this is how a child comes to understand how to move his or her body to create actions or have an effect on his or her environment. This is also how he or she creates an understanding of sensory characteristics, such as sights, sounds, and motions. Examples of exploratory play include playing with rattles, balls, blocks, mobiles, squeeze toys, and small puzzles.

In symbolic play, the child begins to understand how objects are used and how they can control and manipulate objects to create action or change. Primarily through gross motor activities—such as playing with dough, finger painting, puzzles, tumbling, riding a tricycle, or playing on swings (Figure 2-11)—children learn how to move and formulate concepts about the world around them. Simple art activities such as coloring or the use of chalk, glue, or beads to string are just a few examples of the emergence of fine motor activities in play. Interactions with others may also be part of symbolic play, assisting with language development and understanding human relationships. This type of play begins at age 1 year and continues to develop up to age 5 years (Knox, 2005).

Constructive play occurs when the child begins to utilize objects to build and create. Materials used for this type of play range from crayons and paper; activities may include baking cookies or stringing beads (Figure 2-12). This is also termed *creative play*, as this is when imagination and creative expression come to the fore. Creative and constructive play typically begin at age 4 to 7 years (Morrison, Metzger, & Pratt, 1996).

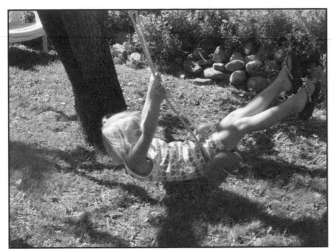

Figure 2-11. Example of child engaged in symbolic play.

Pretend play begins to occur during the second year; it continues and increases up to age 7 years, at which point it begins to taper off (Munier, Myers, & Pierce, 2008). This type of play involves the child imitating or mimicking actions that may or may not occur in the real world. For example, a child may tie a towel around his or her neck, creating a cape and imagining and acting as if he or she were a superhero. Playing with dolls and pretending to cook or prepare a tea party are examples of pretend play. Children often imitate sounds that they believe are created during the action that occurs, such as the sounds cars or trucks make when racing and then crashing into each other.

Children aged 7 to 12 years play games with distinct rules. These games require social interaction and have consequences to actions. They can include structured games such as checkers, card games, or jump rope. Unstructured play activities that have social rules, such as cooking or pet care, are also considered games with rules. The creation of specific objects that require following directions—such as creating arts and crafts objects or models—also falls under this type of play, as it requires following rules in order to complete tasks. Peers, parents, or other adults facilitate the development of rules and social interaction during these activities (Knox, 2005).

Play Participation

"Participating in play; maintaining a balance of play with other areas of occupation; and obtaining, using, and maintaining, toys, equipment, and supplies appropriately" (AOTA, 2014, p. S21).

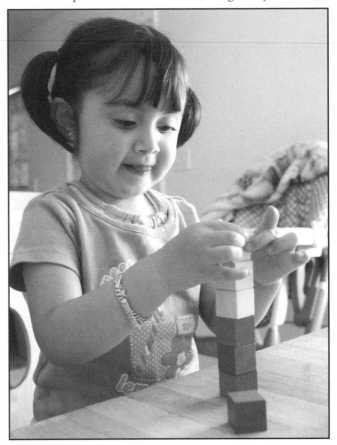

Figure 2-12. Example of a child engaged in constructive play.

Engaging in play is part of human development, facilitating the development of the cognitive, perceptual, and physical skills needed by a mature adult. Without an adequate opportunity to participate in play, a child will not be able to develop the skills that emerge from engaging in play. For example, if a child has little or no contact with other children for the first 6 years of life, he or she will not learn the social skills necessary to socialize with others. Thus, engagement in play is essential to a child's life and must be balanced with other occupations that fill the day.

Play activities are defined by the child or adult participating in them and the environment and culture that surround them. Thus, the variety of activities comprised by play is wide-ranging and diverse. Play activities require varying levels of physical, mental, and social engagement, utilizing a range of objects, toys, and equipment. For one child, play may include making army men out of sticks, while another might use a computer to play video games. Play participation includes the activities involved in obtaining and properly utilizing the objects used in play activities. In some play activities, the child will manipulate an object or the environment, such as shaking a rattle or digging in dirt.

The maintenance of toys and other objects used during play is considered part of the play experience. In order to participate in the play activity, the child must not only gain access to materials or objects, but must also maintain possession of the objects in order to continue playing. For example, if a child is engaged in painting but decides to pour the paint into the toilet, the play activity of painting cannot continue. Understanding how to maintain toys, equipment, and supplies in order to continue play activities emerges after a child has developed the concepts of cause and effect and insight.

Leisure

"A nonobligatory activity that is intrinsically motivated and engaged in during discretionary time, that is time not committed to obligatory occupations such as work, self-care, or sleep (Parham & Fazio, 1997, p. 250)" (AOTA, 2014, p. S21).

How leisure is different from play is a debate seen in the literature for decades. There are more similarities between the two than differences. Play activities are different from leisure in that play is a vital aspect of child development, while leisure is not related to human development in children or adults (Deitz & Swinth, 2008). However, leisure activities are intrinsically motivating to participate in, meaning that there is some emotional reward (which may include enjoyment, entertainment, amusement, or diversion). The most defining aspect of leisure is that it is a nonobligatory activity, which means that it is not an activity that addresses other needs in life. Leisure activity is pursued simply for enjoyment or to meet other intrinsic needs.

Leisure Exploration

"Identifying interests, skills, opportunities, and appropriate leisure activities" (AOTA, 2014, p. S21).

Leisure exploration is the process of finding activities that meet intrinsic needs and that are not obligatory with regard to other aspects of living (such as self-care, child care, home maintenance, etc.). Identifying activities requires seeking out a match of a person's interests, intrinsic needs, and abilities to leisure opportunities. A person who is seeking out leisure opportunities will learn about possible activities by talking to others, watching the activity, watching information about the activity on the television, or searching the Internet. Exploring activities does not necessarily lead to participation. For example, a person may spend time investigating how to take sky diving lessons but find that the personal expense (and fright) outweighs the personal benefits and choose not to follow through with the idea.

Leisure Participation

"Planning and participating in appropriate leisure activities; maintaining a balance of leisure activities with other areas of occupation; and obtaining, using, and maintaining equipment and supplies as appropriate" (AOTA, 2014, p. S21).

As discussed earlier, leisure pursuits are defined as those activities that comprise nonobligatory time and are intrinsically rewarding. How we choose to spend our spare time (discretionary time) is unique to each individual and changes over the life span. Think about the activities you engaged in when you were in high school that you considered fun outside of the educational setting (not related to school). You may still engage in some of these activities, while you may have discarded others for new ones as you matured. Participating in leisure activities is an important part of living a balanced life, regardless of physical or mental abilities or age. Allowing for an adequate balance of time to engage in leisure activities may become difficult because of busy schedules, limited income, or restrictive environment (as in the case of those in prisons or the homeless).

Leisure activities range from active to quiet or sedentary activities. Active activities are those that require active movement within the environment or outdoors. Hiking, shopping, gardening, bike riding, and swimming are just a few examples of active leisure activities. Quiet or sedentary activities are those that require little motor movement and may be done sitting or with small amounts of walking. Examples of sedentary leisure activities are reading, surfing the Internet, watching television, or knitting. Each type provides its own intrinsic rewards, such as happiness, excitement, pride, or self-efficacy. Complete Activity 2-6 to get an idea of what motivates you toward participation in leisure activities.

ACTIVITY 2-6

Think about the activities that you do in your spare time, which do not include ADL, IADL, or other obligatory occupations (those activities that you must do). Next to each activity, describe in a few words how participating in this activity makes you feel. This should also reflect why you chose to participate in the activity.

ACTIVITY	REWARDS

Participating in leisure activities also requires adequate preparation by preparing the self, environment, and objects used. For example, before going to play volleyball, one must first determine where to play volleyball and how to get there. The objects needed must be gathered, such as a ball, other players, water, snacks, and net (if needed). The person will also prepare him- or herself by donning the appropriate clothing and shoes (Figure 2-13). Preparing the body for a hike may also include applying insect repellent or sunscreen. All of these preparatory activities are part of leisure, as they are not linked to other obligatory activities.

Maintaining the equipment and objects used during the leisure activity is also part of participation, as, again, it is not linked to other obligatory occupations and allows for future leisure participation. In other words, assuring that equipment and supplies are kept in usable condition allows the person to use the equipment again in the future. For example, when Vern goes golfing, he cleans each of the golf clubs and puts them back into their proper place once he is done. He cleans the spikes in his golf shoes and puts all of the tees away. This way, when he wants to go golfing again, he has all of the equipment he needs and it will be in working order.

Social Participation

"The interweaving of occupations to support desired engagement in community and family activities as well as those involving peers and friends" (Gillen & Boyt Schell, 2014, p. 607).

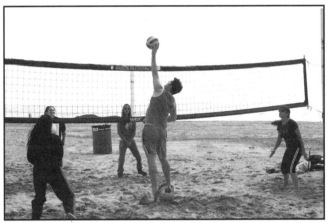

Figure 2-13. Volleyball as an example of a leisure activity.

Involvement in a subset of activities that involve social situations with others (Bedell, 2012) and support social interdependence (Magasi & Hammel, 2004). Social participation can occur in person or through remote technologies such as the telephone, computer interaction, and video conferencing" (AOTA, 2014, p. S21).

Community

"Engaging in activities that result in successful interaction at the community level (i.e., neighborhood, organizations, workplace, school, religious or spiritual group)" (AOTA, 2014, p. S21).

Social interactions at a community level are those that connect two or more individuals as a group. Communities of people are found in many arenas

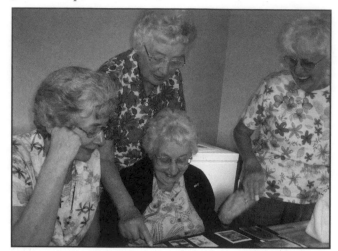

Figure 2-14. An example of sisters going through family pictures as family social participation.

outside of the home, such as at school, at work, within the neighborhood, or possibly at church or in other organizations. Social participation includes not only verbally communicating, but also engaging in activities together. The interactions that occur and that are required to be part of vary according to the social rules of the group. Topics of conversation and how a person acts around others are parts of the social rules that are embedded in the activities surrounding social participation. Socially interacting with others may include physical interactions, such as a hug when meeting, or sharing equipment or objects. Interaction can also occur when one is not face to face with others. Online communities and e-mail are part of community-based social participation, in which there is a very different set of expectations than when interacting in person. Interacting with a person or a group within an online community may include rules such as not using obscene language or pictures, not using all capital letters when writing a sentence, and responding to others in a respectful manner.

Social participation on a community level is different from that at the family or peer level. For example, Jenny participates socially with her coworkers on a level that is different from that with her friends. During breaks and lunches, she and her coworkers joke about their clients and their struggles from the day, while lightly touching on personal topics. Jenny uses terms that her coworkers are familiar with, as they all work in the public relations business. Jenny also will attend after-work events to further the bond with her coworkers, such as attending a beach bonfire party. While Jenny

may refer to some of the people she interacts with as "friends," they are all coworkers, and the social activities, which are work-related, are at a community level.

Family

"Engaging in activities that result in successful interaction in specific required and/or desired familial roles (Mosey, 1996, p. 340)" (AOTA, 2014, p. S21).

Activities involving family interactions are often embedded in culture and tradition (Figure 2-14). Each family will have its own expectations for communication and interaction based on each individual's role within the family. A son may interact with his father differently than with his mother, based on the expectations within his family. Social interaction between family members can occur one-on-one or as a group and does not necessarily occur in person. Just as with social participation within a community, social participation within families can occur via the Internet or phone. Social interactions with family members often surround daily activities such as meal preparation, child rearing, and self-feeding. If one is living with family members, social participation may occur throughout all activities that include the home environment. A child who has many siblings will need to engage socially with his or her brothers and sisters continuously as he or she engages in self-care, play, and possibly educational occupations. Children must communicate their needs, share objects and space, and physically interact with their siblings throughout many of these activities.

Jun is 34 years old and engages in a variety of social activities, each dependent on her familial role. As a daughter, she calls her mom every morning to see how she is feeling and if she needs her to pick up anything from the store. She then wakes up her 4-year-old daughter, singing to her. She wakes up her 2-year-old son by giving him big hugs and tickling him. When she sees her father, she greets him with a hug and a kiss; her interactions with him are filled with respect, and she often turns to him for advice and wisdom. The conversations she has with each of her family members is unique and has its own set of physical interactions. The example of Jun is only a glimpse into how one family interacts. How each family interacts and engages in activities together develops over time and is different for each family unit.

Peer, Friend

"Engaging in activities at different levels of interaction and intimacy, including engaging in desired sexual activity" (AOTA, 2014, p. S21).

Engaging socially with our friends, peers, lovers, and acquaintances occurs in many avenues of our lives and in many different ways. We might engage in small talk about the weather with an acquaintance or someone we just met at a party, while we might cry on the shoulder of a good friend and talk of our deepest woes. Engaging with others occurs not only in the community, workplace, and within family groups, but also in solitary relationships with those who we see as peers. Activities involving social participation with friends or peers often occur within other occupations, such as talking with a friend while shopping or sharing a joke while riding on a ski lift. Engagement in social activities is reflected in interactions between two people, how their bodies move in relation to each other, and sharing the experience of engaging in an occupation together. The occupations can be very intimate, such as sexual activity, or purely platonic, such as sharing a meal together. The type of relationship existing between two people determines the intensity and level of social participation. It is the engagement in social activities that establishes, maintains, or destroys the relationship. Friendships are developed by engaging in conversations and shared experiences. The friendship is maintained by the respective participants' actions, with continued action involving both participants. For example, Mercedes and Alison met at a mutual friend's party. They began talking about their children and found that they had much in common. At the end of the evening, they exchanged e-mail addresses (Figure 2-15). Shortly thereafter, they met for coffee. Now they call or e-mail each other once a week and occasionally go for a walk or meet for breakfast. The actions Alison took to connect with Mercedes, and those taken by Mercedes to become friends with Alison, were all social participation activities.

OCCUPATION AWARENESS

In conducting an occupation-based activity analysis, in order to gain an understanding of the meaning behind an activity that has meaning to your client (an occupation), it is important to gather information regarding how your client defines that occupation.

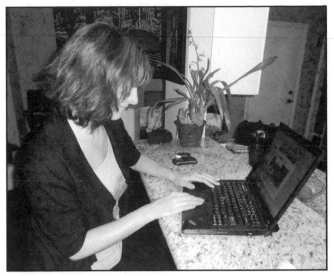

Figure 2-15. Socializing often occurs within the virtual context.

The first half of this chapter was dedicated to defining the areas of occupation as they are listed in the *Framework*. There were multiple activities and tasks listed under the areas of ADL, IADL, rest and sleep, education, work, play, leisure, and social participation. As you may recall, some activities may be classified into several different areas of occupation based on how the client defines them. For example, painting can be seen as a leisure activity or as work, based on why the client is painting. The first best step to an occupation-based activity analysis is asking the client to define the occupation he or she wants or needs to do. What defines successful participation for him or her? How does this occupation play a part in his or her life?

Understanding the occupation also requires understanding the person participating in the occupation—gaining knowledge of his or her values, beliefs, and spirituality. Values are defined as "acquired beliefs and commitments, derived from culture, about what is good, right and important to do (Kielhofner, 2008)" (AOTA, 2014, p. S22). Beliefs are "cognitive content held as true to the client" (AOTA, 2014, p. S22). Beliefs and values influence how and why a person performs an occupation. A person who does not believe in using electricity to cook may perform cooking tasks differently. Values influence the standards to which a person will hold when a decision must be made during an activity or the emphasis they put on efforts toward certain steps. A person who values family may put a great amount of effort into including all members of the family in an ancestry scrapbook. The spirituality of the person and the spiritual meaning the occupation has for the client can influence performance as well. Spirituality is related to "the aspect of humanity that refers to the way individuals seek and express meaning and purpose and the way they experience their connectedness to the moment, to self, to others, to nature, and to the significant or sacred" (Puchalski et al., 2009, p. 887). The guiding motivations to act during an occupation may come from spiritual motivation, derived meaning beyond money or tangible benefits. For example, a client may choose to volunteer at a homeless shelter because of the spiritual meaning it has for him or her, giving him or her a sense of purpose and fulfillment.

CONCLUSION

Determining what to analyze and paring it down to a workable activity is the first step to activity analysis (see Activity 2-2). This requires having an understanding of what defines success for the client or as the activity is typically done if conducting a standard activity analysis. The *Framework* has helped clinicians to define occupations and the scope of our practice by creating major categories of occupations and defining what activities fit into each of those categories through the "Areas of Occupation" section of the *Framework*. This can be used in activity analysis to help the clinician define in what area of occupation the activity is classified, as well as to clarify all of the tasks that are part of the activity.

Defining which area of occupation is being analyzed requires the practitioner to gather information from the client about how he or she defines the occupation. This information is gathered in the Occupational Profile. During this interview, the practitioner should also gather information regarding the meaning and importance of the occupation. This will be discussed in the next chapter.

QUESTIONS

1. What is the purpose of the Areas of Occupation section of the *Framework*?
2. How is "feeding" different from "eating"?
3. What is the difference between a prosthetic and an orthotic? How are these part of the ADL?
4. Why is sleep listed as an occupation?

5. What are ways in which community mobility is conducted?
6. What are at least three activities that would be considered part of retirement preparation?
7. What activities would be considered play if an adult was the participant?
8. List three social participation activities.
9. How do occupations give our lives meaning?

ACTIVITIES

1. Complete the first step of the activity analysis process for an occupation you enjoy engaging in. (1) Name the occupation, being as specific as possible as to clarify what defines success. (2) Identify which area of occupation the activity or occupation lies in (if an occupation-based analysis, the category will depend on how the client defines the occupation). (3) If conducting an occupation-based analysis, describe the relevance and importance of the occupation to you.
2. What is the range of occupations in which humans engage? Using a variety of magazines, cut out pictures of people engaging in occupations. As a class, create eight poster boards, one for each area of occupation. The class can divide up into groups, each addressing an area of occupation. Once completed, share each board—the visual representation of the broad spectrum of activities that are included in each area. Collectively, all of these boards represent the domain of OT and can be displayed for others to see.
3. Create a list of occupations that define who you are. Using that list, create a visual representation of yourself as an occupational being.
4. Complete Activity 2-7.
5. For each of the following case studies, do the following:
   a. Identify each of the activities/occupations with which the client is having difficulties and indicate the area of occupation into which each belongs according to the Framework.
   b. Prepare a list of other examples of activities that are included in the areas of occupation you identified in the case study.

ACTIVITY 2-7

Indicate which area(s) of occupation each activity or task would be categorized as:

	ADL	IADL	EDUC-ATION	WORK	PLAY	LEISURE	SOCIAL PAR-TICIPATION
Surf the web							
Organize your CD collection							
Ride a bike							
Fold laundry							
Pour a cup of coffee							
Sing in the shower							
Write a paper for an OT class							
Put on ski boots							
Throw a party							
Put gas in the car							
Get newspaper from yard							
Cut coupons							
Take a bubble bath							
Smoke a cigarette							
Go to church							
Water plants							
Pick lint out of belly button							

The purpose of this exercise was to get you thinking about the different areas of occupation and being able to identify which categories different activities might fall under. There is also another hidden objective behind this activity. Compare your answers to some of your classmates' answers. Are they different? Why? This exercise shows how the meaning behind occupations can be different for each individual. For example, I consider organizing a CD collection as an IADL, as home establishment and management (it is not a fun task for me). However, if you asked my husband, he would consider this leisure as well. He enjoys doing this, and painstakingly alphabetizes each CD with glee. It is a requirement of home establishment and management but also has leisure aspects for him. If I asked you to categorize the activity of painting a picture, would you consider that leisure? As an OT student, it could be leisure or part of a class and thus classified under "formal education participation." But let's say you have a client who is a professional artist. Painting is now considered work. Thus, the areas of occupation are best utilized when conducting occupation-based activity analyses (within the contexts of an individual).

Joey

Joey is a 10-year-old boy with autism who has been referred to you for OT. His mother reports that he has been having difficulty with tasks at home and at school. His mother is concerned about the fact that he does not have any friends. He only enjoys playing video games and does not engage in any other activities that other boys of his age usually do. His parents signed him up for a karate class, but he does not engage with the instructor or follow the directions given in class. His mother reports very proudly that he is now able to dress himself but has difficulty picking out appropriate clothing. He will occasionally have "accidents" when he does not get to the bathroom to urinate and soils his clothing.

Connie

Connie is a 73-year-old woman who has just moved to the assisted living facility where you work. She has moved there because her husband recently passed away and she was living alone and needed assistance. She reports to you that she is very lonely and feels that since her husband passed away, she rarely sees her family. She says she used to be so active but is now bored. She would like to do something with her time but is not sure what to do. She spends all day in her apartment with her cat. She says she would like to be able to go to church on Sundays but is unable to drive herself there (her husband used to drive them both to church).

Upon visiting her in her new apartment, you see that the living area is full of clutter and is messy. There is a large stack of mail sitting on her table, which she says consists mostly of bills that she has not paid (her husband used to handle all of the bills). There is a litter box in the bathroom, which appears to not have been cleaned in a very long time.

Matt

Matt, age 24 years, was recently admitted to the rehabilitation hospital where you work. He suffered a traumatic brain injury while snowboarding without a helmet and was in a coma for 2 weeks. He is severely cognitively limited in motor planning and memory. His right side is paralyzed, and he is right-hand dominant. He uses a wheelchair to move around the unit but runs into objects on his right side. When he eats his meals, he often misses the food that is on the right side of his plate. He is able to indicate when he needs to go to the bathroom but is not able to wipe himself thoroughly.

He expresses that he wants to leave the hospital and will often try to stand up by himself; thus he has fallen twice. The nurses report that he is up most of the night. He naps throughout the day. Matt had been a construction worker, in charge of putting up drywall in new homes. He and his family are worried that he will lose his job. Matt's primary worry is whether he will be able to return to snowboarding. He and his girlfriend were planning on getting married and

having children soon. He worries that she won't stay with him, as they have not had any time alone together in a long while.

Gina

Gina, age 32 years, recently lost both arms at the elbow in an explosion at work. Gina worked in the chemistry department of a university as a lab assistant. She has a 9-month-old baby at home. She is worried about how she will feed and bathe the baby once she goes home. She has two prosthetic arms but is unable to put them on herself. She has been unable to clean her contact lenses, so she has been wearing glasses. She would like to be able to call her husband and family but must ask nurses to place the call for her and they must stand and hold the phone against her ear.

She tells you that she has difficulties at night, as she usually likes to listen to her iPod to help her go to sleep, but she has been unable to do this. She also likes to wash her face and remove all her makeup before she goes to bed but cannot do so by herself. She is embarrassed to say that she must ask her husband or nurses to help her put on her makeup in the morning.

She does not want to return to her previous job, but is interested in finding another line of work. She is not sure what she would like to do. She was also very active in sports activities and is not sure what she will be able to return to.

Norman

Norman is 41 years old and has been referred to OT in an outpatient psychiatric unit. He has obsessive-compulsive disorder, as well as PTSD from a tour of duty in Iraq several years earlier. He is also a recovering alcoholic. He has not been taking his medication for anxiety; therefore, his symptoms have become worse. His case manager has notified you that Norman has accrued extensive credit card debt from buying things online and is now struggling to be able to buy his food.

Norman reports that when he does buy food, he buys junk food and does not make healthy meals for himself. Norman feels that he must always be busy and does not stop to rest during the day, leaving him feeling exhausted by nightfall. He stays busy by working out at the gym and cleaning his house, even if he just finished cleaning it. There is an Alcoholics Anonymous

(AA) group for veterans that meets in his neighborhood, but he has been nervous about attending and has never gone. The leader of the group has contacted him several times to see if he would volunteer to be a sponsor for new AA members. Norman would like to do this.

REFERENCES

American Occupational Therapy Association. (2014). Occupational therapy practice framework: Domain and process (3rd ed.). *American Journal of Occupational Therapy, 68*(Suppl.1), S1-S48.

Billock, C. (2009). Spirituality, occupation, and occupational therapy. In E. Crepeau, E. Cohn, & B. Boyt Schell (Eds.). *Willard and Spackman's occupational therapy* (11th ed., pp. 90-96). Philadelphia, PA: Lippincott Williams & Wilkins.

Billock, C. (2014). Personal values, beliefs, and spirituality. In B. Boyt Schell, G. Gillen, & M. Scaffa (Eds.). *Willard and Spackman's occupational therapy* (12th ed., pp. 225-231). Baltimore, MD: Lippincott Williams & Wilkins.

Christiansen, C. H. (1999). Defining lives: Occupation as identity: An essay on competence, coherence, and the creation of meaning, 1999 Eleanor Clarke Slagle lecture. *American Journal of Occupational Therapy, 53*, 547-558.

Christiansen, C., & Hammecker, C. (2001). Self care. In B. R. Bonder & M. B. Wagner (Eds.), Functional performance in older adults (pp. 155-715). Philadelphia, PA: F. A. Davis.

Cook, A., & Hussey, S. (2002). *Assistive technologies: Principles and practice* (2nd ed.). St. Louis, MO: Mosby.

Cook, A., & Polgar, F. (2008). *Cook & Hussey's Assistive Technologies* (3rd ed.). St. Louis, MO: Mosby Elsevier.

Dave, D., Rashad, I., & Spasojevic, J. (2008). The effects of retirement on physical and mental health outcomes. *Southern Economic Journal, 75*(2), 497-524.

Deitz, J., & Swinth, Y. (2008). Accessing play through assistive technology. In L. D. Parham, & L. Fazio (Eds.), *Play in occupational therapy for children* (2nd ed., pp. 395-412). St. Louis, MO: Mosby Elsevier.

Deshaies, L. (2008). Upper extremity orthoses. In M. Radomski & C. Trombly Latham (Eds.), *Occupational therapy for physical dysfunction* (6th ed., pp. 421-464). Baltimore, MD: Lippincott Williams & Wilkins.

Hagedorn, R. (1995). *Occupational therapy, perspectives and processes*. Edinburgh, UK: Churchill Livingstone.

Hagedorn, R. (1997). *Foundations for practice in occupational therapy*. Edinburgh, UK: Churchill Livingstone.

Hinojosa, J., Kramer, P., & Pratt, P. (1996). Foundations of practice: Developmental principles, theories, and frames of reference. In J. Case-Smith, A. Allen, & P. Pratt (Eds.), *Occupational therapy for children* (3rd ed., pp. 25-45). St. Louis, MO: Mosby.

Knox, S. (2005). Play. In J. Case-Smith (Ed.), *Occupational therapy for children* (5th ed., pp. 571-586). St. Louis, MO: Mosby Elsevier.

McKnight-Eily, L., Presley-Cantrell, L., Strine, T., Chapman, D., Perry, G., & Croft, J. (2008). Perceived insufficient rest or sleep—Four states. *Morbidity and Mortality Weekly, 57*(8), 200-203.

McMinn, A. (2009). Active retirement for healthier aging. *Perspectives in Public Health, 129*(4), 158-160.

Moriera-Almeida, A., & Koenig, H. G. (2006). Retaining the meaning of the words religiousness and spirituality: A commentary on the WHOQOL SRPB group's "A cross-cultural study of spirituality, religion, and personal beliefs as components of quality of life." *Social Science and Medicine, 62*(6), 843-844.

Morrison, C., Metzger, P., & Pratt, P. (1996). Play. In J. Case-Smith, A. Allen, & P. Pratt (Eds.), *Occupational therapy for children* (3rd ed., pp. 504-524). St. Louis, MO: Mosby.

Mosby's dictionary of medicine, nursing & health professions. (2006). St. Louis, MO: Mosby Elsevier.

Mosey, A. (1996). *Applied scientific inquiry in the health professions: An epistemological orientation* (2nd ed.). Bethesda, MD: American Occupational Therapy Association.

Moyers, P., & Dale, L. (2007). *The guide to occupational therapy practice* (2nd ed.). Bethesda, MD: AOTA Press.

Munier, V., Myers, C., & Pierce, D. (2008). Power of object play for infants and toddlers. In L. D. Parham & L. Fazio (Eds.), *Play in occupational therapy for children* (2nd ed., pp. 219-249). St. Louis, MO: Mosby Elsevier.

Nurit, W., & Michel, A. (2003). Rest: A qualitative exploration of the phenomenon. *Occupational Therapy International, 10*, 227-238.

Parham, L. D. (2008). Play and occupational therapy. In L. D. Parham & L. Fazio (Eds.), *Play in occupational therapy for children* (2nd ed., pp. 3-39). St. Louis, MO: Mosby Elsevier.

Parham, L., & Fazio, L. (Eds.). (1997). *Play in occupational therapy for children.* St. Louis, MO: Mosby.

Puchalski, C., Ferrell, B., Virani, R., Otis-Green, S., Baird, P., Bull, J.,...Sulmasy, D. (2009). Improving the quality of spiritual care as a dimension of palliative care: The report of the Consensus Conference. *Journal of Palliative Medicine, 12*, 885-904.

Rogers, J., & Holm, M. (1994). Assessment of self-care. In B. R. Bonder & M. B. Wagner (Eds.), *Functional performance in older adults* (pp. 181-202). Philadelphia, PA: F. A. Davis.

West, L. (2009). Sleep: An emerging practice area? *OT Practice, 14*(8), 9-10.

Wilcock, A. (1993). A theory of the human need for occupation. *Journal of Occupational Science: Australia, 1*(1), 17-24.

World Health Organization. (2001). *International classification of functioning, disability, and health.* Geneva, Switzerland: Author.

STEPS TO ACTIVITY ANALYSIS

Step 1: Determine What Is Being Analyzed
Chapter 2

Step 2: Determine the Relevance and Importance to the Client
Chapter 3

Step 3: Determine the Sequence and Timing
Chapter 4

Step 4: Determine Object, Space, and Social Demands
Chapter 5

Step 5: Determine Required Body Functions
Chapter 6

Step 6: Determine Required Body Structures
Chapter 7

Step 7: Determine Required Actions and Performance Skills
Chapter 8

3

Step 2: Determine the Relevance and Importance to the Client

Occupation-Based Activity Analysis

Objectives

- Understand which aspects of the client are key to conducting an occupation-based activity analysis.
- Identify how the client's values, beliefs, and spirituality influence participation in occupations and activities.
- List the information gathered during an occupational profile.
- Explain how the client's physical, social, cultural, personal, temporal, and virtual contexts can influence his or her performance in occupations and activities.
- Understand how performance patterns such as habits, routines, rituals, and roles all influence participation in occupations and activities.

Activities can be examined from the perspective of the typical demands of an activity or with the client's perspective or contexts in mind. Activities themselves do not lie in isolation but are woven into individual lives with distinct features and demands based on the physical and social environment within which the person performs the activity. In order to understand the demands of an activity as a client needs and wants to do it, an occupation-based activity analysis must be completed. This chapter focuses on the unique characteristics of occupation-based activity analysis and how it is conducted. It also examines the contexts that support or inhibit participation in the occupation. This includes examining the cultural, personal, temporal, virtual, physical, and social contexts. The client's interests, values, beliefs, and spirituality also influence elements of participation. Performance patterns, such as the habits, routines, rituals, and roles, may also play an important part in the occupation being studied.

Activity Demands Redefined

In order to understand how an occupation is defined by a client, each of the activity demands of the occupation the client needs or wants to do must be examined, as well as how they manifest within the client's life. In order to do this, the process in which the activity analysis is conducted is slightly different, in that instead of understanding just an activity, you are becoming aware of the client and how he or

Thomas H.
Occupation-Based Activity Analysis, Second Edition (pp 45-55).
© 2015 SLACK Incorporated.

she defines an occupation. As we move forward in the activity analysis process, you will find that there are aspects of an activity that, if changed, change the person's performance requirements. For example, if the handle of the toothbrush is very narrow, the joint mobility of the user's fingers must be very good. However, if we increase the width of handle, like the handles of many electric toothbrushes, the user's finger joints will not have to be quite so mobile. Thus it is important for us to know the properties of the different objects our clients use when they engage in the occupation we are analyzing. Understanding these objects and their properties is just one aspect of the activity analysis process. We must aware of this as we conduct an occupation-based activity analysis.

RELEVANCE AND IMPORTANCE

Determining Relevance and Importance

There is an abundance of literature in the OT profession that speaks to the concepts surrounding occupations and meaning. Human beings engage in daily activities that give their lives meaning and serve a purpose. We define ourselves by what we do. It is through our occupations that we experience life's meaning (Christiansen, 1999; Crabtree, 1998). Each occupation we engage in carries a different meaning in our lives and has a unique value. The meaning and importance of each occupation is defined by our clients' goals, values, beliefs, and needs and the perceived utility of their occupations.

Values are defined as "acquired beliefs and commitments, derived from culture, about what is good, right and important to do (Kielhofner, 2008)" (AOTA, 2014, p. S22). Beliefs are "cognitive content held as true to the client" (AOTA, 2014, p. S22). For example, a person can highly value honesty, commitment, hard work, and independence. These values will influence the meaning that a given occupation has for the client. George, a client in a drug and alcohol rehabilitation center, expresses that he wants to be able to regain a solid, healthy relationship with his wife. When questioned further, he explains that he will not be able to go home to his wife until he is sober. He strongly values his marriage and states that he will do anything to maintain his commitment to his wife. The values

George holds regarding marriage give us valuable information regarding the occupations of sexual activity and social participation.

Beliefs comprise the cognitive content that a client holds as true (AOTA, 2014, p. S22). For example, a person might believe that all hard work pays off or that fate determines our future. These beliefs often influence a client's determination or perspective on his or her future and how much influence he or she has in determining outcomes. Some belief systems are culturally based. For example, a client might believe that he has become ill because of the bad actions of someone in his family or his past. Therefore, he may believe that the illness or disability is a burden that he must bear. Conversely, some might believe that all challenges can be overcome with hard work. Understanding your client's beliefs regarding his occupations and current performance will clarify his definition of the occupations you are analyzing, as well as give some ideas about how intervention could be approached.

Each occupation a person engages in serves a specific need or utility. Survival and meeting basic bodily needs are foundational to much of what we do every day. However, in addition to providing for our basic needs (food, shelter, self-care), we used occupations to develop skills, meet personal needs, and establish superiority over those who might be seen as predatory (Wilcock, 1993). Some researchers have found that people use occupations to pass on information to children, establish order in families or households (Segal, 1999), or express individual skill or pride (De Vault, 1991; Miller, 1998). These are just a few examples of the range of needs that are met through occupations.

The needs that are met by an occupation are uniquely defined by each client, although most clients may be unaware of them until they are questioned. For example, Carmen is a client in an outpatient hand therapy clinic. During the evaluation, she identifies several occupations as important for her to return to. One of them is washing dishes, which she has not been able to do since she broke her wrist. When asked to explain the importance of this occupation, she had to sit and think about why this was so important to her. She stated, "I guess I just really like to have the house clean when my husband comes home, and to be honest, it is a really relaxing activity for me. I like the feel of the warm water and soap and the look of the shiny dishes when I am done." This says so much about her values and the needs that this occupation fulfills for Carmen. She feels that she needs to do it for her husband (also a value), but she also uses this activity to help her relax.

To determine the relevance and importance of an activity and to determine the client's values, beliefs, and needs, as well as the perceived utility of an occupation, consider asking the client the following questions:

- In what ways is this activity important to you?
- How does engaging in this activity make you feel?
- In what ways do you need to engage in this activity?
- Tell me about the experiences you have when engaged in this activity.
- How has limited ability to engage in this activity affected your life? Your roles? Your relationships with others?
- How does this activity define who you are? (Hocking, 2001)

Defining the Occupation

How your client defines an occupation gives you important information regarding the relevance that this occupation has in his or her life as well as some insight into how important that occupation is to the client. In Chapter 2, the areas of occupation were defined as they are listed in the *Framework*. Multiple activities and tasks were listed under the areas of ADL, IADL, rest and sleep, education, work, play, leisure, and social participation. As you may recall, some activities may be classified into several different areas of occupation based on how the client defines them. For example, painting can be seen as a leisure activity or as work based on why the client is painting. The first best step to an occupation-based activity analysis is asking the client to define the occupation he or she wants or needs to do. What defines successful participation for him or her? How does this occupation play a part in his or her life?

Perceived Utility

The OT literature provides a broad range of perspectives on how the meaning behind occupations drives our identities. A commonly held belief in our profession is that the occupations that we engage in define who we are. This concept of "occupational identity" relates to this concept and how a person's values, interests, and roles are integrated (Hocking, 2001). If you think about it, as human beings, our daily existence consists of engaging in one occupation after another. The occupations in which we choose to engage define who we are. Think about what you have done today, from the time you woke up to right now. How many of those activities fulfill a role of which you are part? Reading this book is part of your role as a student. What activities do you engage in that are part of how you define yourself? If you were suddenly no longer able to engage in those activities, would you lose your sense of self? Thinking of occupations from this perspective, as being part of a person's identity, can help you better analyze the demands of the activity or occupation your client wishes to engage in.

In addition to understanding the meaning behind an occupation, it is also very important to understand what function or purpose is served by engaging in the occupation. Humans engage in occupations for a wide variety of reasons: to meet bodily needs, to maintain shelter, for social sustenance, and for internal gratification. Research has explored the numerous reasons why people engage in occupations, the findings of which could comprise another book. For the purpose of this book, it is important to understand that as we strive to fully analyze every element of an occupation, we must gain perspective on what purpose the occupation serves for our client. It may be easy for us to attach our own values and beliefs about what purpose an occupation serves, but this could lead to an inaccurate analysis. For example, we might assume that our client Shira attends temple services on Saturdays because of her deep spiritual beliefs. However, after interviewing Shira, we find that the perceived utility of going to services is to try to find a husband "of good character" (as she states it). As the utility of the occupation is defined by Shira, the demands of the activity and how it takes place differ (perhaps she dresses and acts differently than if the purpose were for something other than finding a future husband).

Occupation-Based Activity Analysis: Understanding the Form of the Occupation

As we move forward in the activity analysis process, we will learn about how to analyze the objects and properties, space demands, and social demand of an activity. In conducting an occupation-based activity analysis, the result of each step of the analysis will be unique to the client. The objects used will be unique to the individual, as will the way he or she performs the activity, with whom it is performed, and where it is performed. It is important to remember that we must gain a full understanding of what the occupation looks like. As with the example given in Chapter 1 of making a peanut butter and jelly sandwich, the same activity may look different when a different client is performing it. The demands on the participant change as the objects, space, and social demands change.

Let's use an example we can all relate to: brushing our teeth. If you were to ask all the people in your class to videotape themselves brushing their teeth, you would find no two people doing the activity in exactly the same way. This is because the objects they would be using are different, their environments are different, and the way they define the activity will be different. Thus, when we work with clients, we cannot assume that the form of an occupation they are speaking of is the same form in which we might do it. You might have a client who states that she wants to be able to brush her teeth but she does this standing in the shower as part of her daily morning routine!

THE OCCUPATIONAL PROFILE

In order to gain an understanding of how a client defines an occupation; the meaning and utility of an occupation; the client's values, beliefs and spirituality; and in what form the occupation takes place, the OT practitioner gathers this information through an occupational profile. The occupational profile is part of the evaluation process but does not necessarily occur only at the initiation of services. The profile is conducted through an interview of the client and the client's family, caregivers, and other significant people in his or her life. The purpose of the profile is to gain an understanding of the client's interests, values, needs, occupational history, patterns of daily living, and his or her priorities for outcomes (AOTA, 2014). Through the process of interviewing the client (and significant others), the OT practitioner should be able to determine the following:

- Why the client is receiving services—what are his or her concerns with daily life activities.
- Which occupation(s) he or she is having trouble with, and which have been successful.

- Which aspects of the client's environment or contexts support or inhibit participation in the occupation(s).
- What occupations the client has participated in the past, what he or she currently engages in, and what desired future occupations are.
- What are the client's values and interests?
- What roles does the client fulfill?
- What are the client's patterns of daily activities—how have these patterns changed?
- What are the client's priorities—what are their desired outcomes? (AOTA, 2014)

There is no set list of questions to ask the client, as the profile is dynamically changing and interactive. The practitioner should actively listen to the client and base questions not only on the needed information, but on the client's responses. Questioning the client about occupations that are difficult will give you a basis on which to break down and analyze the occupation. Within the occupational profile process, information must also be gleaned about the client's environment and contexts, providing valuable information regarding the objects required, space demands, and social demands (Activity 3-1).

ACTIVITY 3-1

List at least four questions to be asked during an occupational profile that would determine:
- How the client defines the occupation being analyzed
- The perceived utility of the occupation
- The values or beliefs that guide participation in the occupation
- The spiritual aspects or components of participation in the occupation

_____

_____

_____

_____

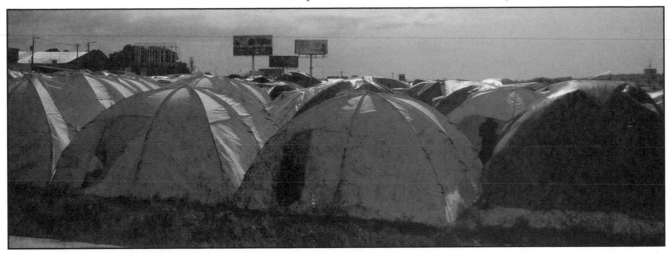

Figure 3-1. An example of how the environment can influence performance: The rubble-filled streets of Haiti impede the residents' ability to navigate their community and conduct business.

CONTEXTS AND ENVIRONMENTS

Contexts and environments are conditions within and around the client, all of which influence performance and are important considerations in analyzing an activity or occupation. The *Framework* uses the terms *environment* and *contexts*. Environments are those elements that surround the client—the physical environment and the social environment. Contexts are those aspects that not only surround the client but are also within the client and influence performance. The *Framework* delineates four contexts: cultural, personal, temporal, and virtual. An understanding of these elements provides information regarding the challenges or demands that the client experiences during performance. These contexts can either support or inhibit participation in an occupation. Developing an understanding of a client's contexts begins with the occupational profile and continues throughout the evaluation and intervention process.

The Physical Environment

The external environment is called the *physical environment* and includes all nonhuman objects and space. It includes both human-made and natural environments. It is important to understand the physical environment in which an occupation occurs, as this can influence the demand for performance skills and body functions. The terrain, temperature, size, noise level, and lighting are all part of the physical context that should be considered as part of the space demands

for the occupation (Figure 3-1). The objects that are part of the environment should also be considered, as their placement, arrangement, and properties can also have an influence on participation. Buildings, plants, tables, tools, equipment, and furniture are examples of objects that are part of the physical context (AOTA, 2014). This information can be utilized to determine the objects and properties required for an occupation, as well as to provide additional information about the objects surrounding the environment in which the occupation takes place (Activity 3-2).

ACTIVITY 3-2

What is part of the physical environment in which you engage in the occupation of studying? (If you have more than one place in which you study, choose one.) Describe all aspects of the environment, as well as the objects in the environment.

The Social Environment

The *social environment* is the "presences, relationships with, and expectations of persons, groups or populations with whom the client has contact" (AOTA, 2014, p. S28). The social environment can include the client's friends, spouse, boyfriend/girlfriend, caregivers, coworkers, colleagues, or associations with organizations or groups of people. It is the availability and expectations of these individuals, groups, or populations that influence norms, role expectations, and social routines. These relationships can provide a support or be a hindrance to participation in occupations. For example, a spouse can support a client's actions toward writing in a journal every day by giving him or her privacy and quiet during the client's writing time. For a client who is trying to stop drinking alcohol, a group of friends can be a hindrance by offering alcoholic drinks to the client. Gaining awareness of the social environments in which the client functions can clarify the social demands of the occupations in which the client needs or wants to engage.

The Cultural Context

The client's customs, behavior standards, activity patterns, and beliefs are shaped by his or her *cultural context* (AOTA, 2014). A client's cultural context influences his or her identity and activity choices (AOTA, 2014). Family traditions are part of the client's culture and determine the roles and expectations of the client's actions. How a person dresses, greets others, and acts toward strangers is set by cultural expectations and can change based on the cultural context. For example, in France people greet each other by kissing each cheek, while in the United States people traditionally shake hands. Within organizations, a specific culture emerges with expectations and actions that are unique. For example, in one hospital there may be an expectation that all occupational therapists address sexuality with their clients, while in another hospital it is the psychologist who does this. Geographic areas may have a culture that determines attitudes and behaviors with the residents. For example, there are distinct cultural differences between residents of California and those of New York (Activity 3-3).

ACTIVITY 3-3

What are some of the cultural beliefs, behavior standards, and expectations of the city or state in which you live? What is the culture of your school?

The Personal Context

The *personal context* involves aspects of the person that are not health-related but are still personal identifiers, such as age, gender, educational level, and socioeconomic status (AOTA, 2014). It is important to understand that disability or diagnosis is not part of the personal context. The personal context can apply to a personal role within an organization and the specific population to which a person belongs. For example, the personal context of a client might be that he is a 62-year-old male who is a part-time employee of a construction company and is a Vietnam veteran. Understanding your client's personal context gives you a better understanding of the demands of the occupations he or she needs to engage in. The client's age may influence the type of occupation, how it is performed, and its complexity. For example, gardening to a 4-year-old may be very different from gardening to a 70-year-old. Socioeconomic level has an impact on multiple aspects of engagement in occupations, primarily access to needed space and objects. For example, a homeless man may have greater difficulty in finding access to a computer to search job openings than would a man of middle income who has a computer in his home. The educational level of the client will reflect in his or her reading ability and access to certain opportunities. A woman without a high school diploma will have limited access to occupations that require a high school diploma or a higher educational level. As with all of the contexts, the personal context can support or inhibit participation in an occupation but can also provide needed information regarding the demands of the occupation (Activity 3-4).

ACTIVITY 3-4

Describe your personal context. This includes your age, gender, socioeconomic group, educational level, and whatever organizational or social status you may have.

The Temporal Context

Occupations occur within a space in time, which is the *temporal context*. Time is defined by stages of life, duration of actual time, time of day, rhythm of activity, or time of year. The temporal context can influence how an occupation is performed, when, and at what pace. For example, if the length of time available for a client to prepare a meal is very short, the demands are very different on the client than if he or she had hours to prepare it. The client's stage of life may also change the demands of the occupation, as paying bills, for example, is very different for those in early adulthood than for those at the end of life. The pattern and rhythm of an occupation contributes to its temporal aspects. This includes the timing of steps, the repetition of certain aspects of the occupation, and how the occupation is woven into a sequence of other occupations. Understanding the temporal context that surrounds and influences the occupation being analyzed allows the clinician to recognize how aspects of timing and placement of the occupation within the spectrum of time can influence the demands on the client. For example, if John typically wakes up at 9 a.m. to leave for work at 9:45 a.m., the clinician has an idea of the time of day when John conducts his self-care as well as the amount of time he has to complete all of the self-care tasks (Activity 3-5).

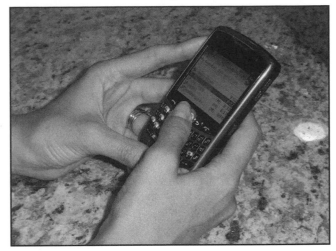

Figure 3-2. The virtual context is used for many daily occupations, including shopping and social participation.

ACTIVITY 3-5

What are the temporal contexts for your morning self-care routine on the days in which you go to school or work? How would the demands of the occupation change if you woke up late and had half the time?

The Virtual Context

Communication occurring by means of airways or computers and in the absence of physical contact occurs in the *virtual context* (AOTA, 2014). This takes place through the use of computers, the Internet, cellular phones, telephones, video conferencing, and radio transmission. The virtual context is an environment in which information can be sent and received without physical interaction with another. This can occur via chat rooms or platforms, e-mail, video conferencing, radio transmissions, remote monitoring via wireless sensors or computer-based data collection (AOTA, 2014). Advancements in technology including portable devices such as cellular phones and tablets have expanded this context to nearly everywhere (Figure 3-2). A client can be supported or inhibited in his or her occupations by access or lack of access to the virtual context. A person who was recently diagnosed with multiple sclerosis can connect with others with the same diagnosis through an online support

group. A father coaching his son's baseball team may be interrupted by e-mail and text messages coming in on his cellular phone. The virtual context may or may not influence a client's desired occupation. Given the current use of technology and its immersion into daily life, the virtual context can be an embedded part of any occupation that the client uses intermittently during another occupation. For example, a client may check her e-mail on her phone periodically while she is cooking dinner (Activity 3-6).

ACTIVITY 3-6

What virtual contexts are part of your daily occupations? What virtual contexts do you embed within other occupations?

PERFORMANCE PATTERNS

Performance patterns are the habits, routines, rituals, and roles that influence and surround participation in occupations. When one is analyzing an occupation, an essential step is to investigate the patterns in which the client engages and how they influence the demands of the occupation. Habits and routines can influence how and when an occupation is performed. This can be found to be either a support or hindrance to performance.

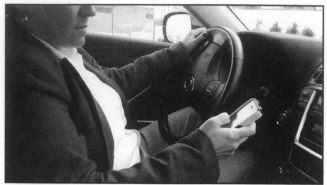

Figure 3-3. Continuous and intrusive use of a cell phone can be a bad habit if it interferes with performance in other occupations, such as driving.

Habits

Habits are "acquired tendencies to respond and perform in certain consistent ways in familiar environments or situations" (AOTA, 2014, p. S27). They are automatic behaviors or action that are performed repeatedly and with little variation and are part of everyday life (AOTA, 2014). Habits allow us to move and function on a more automatic basis. These habits emerge from repetition until the behaviors become automatic. Habits can be useful, dominating, or impoverished. While many habits allow us to function at a higher level and are useful, there are many habits that limit functioning and are termed *dominating*. A useful habit would be to automatically shut and lock the door when leaving the house. A dominating habit would be chewing on fingernails while talking to a stranger or repeatedly washing one's hands. An impoverished habit is a habit that is not fully developed, is lacking in consistency, or has not yet been embedded in the client's daily routines.

Understanding a client's habits will help the clinician understand where in the client's daily routine occupations occur and help to understand where habits may interfere of help with performance. Discovering a client's habits also may help to uncover the steps used to complete an occupation if there are simultaneous occupations occurring, as well as the timing and sequence of these steps. A client's habits may interfere with meeting the demands of the activity or may be a part of successful participation (Figure 3-3; Activity 3-7).

Routines

Routines are also part of performance patterns that occur regularly and provide structure for the flow of

daily activities. Routines are patterns of behavior and actions that are observable and repetitive. A routine can be satisfying, promoting, or damaging. Most routines follow a sequence of actions that are embedded in cultural or ecological contexts (Fiese, 2007; Segal, 2004). For example, before going to bed, many people perform a series of steps in order to prepare themselves for sleep. At the end of the day, when the body and mind are often tired, routines make it easier to complete all of the tasks needed to prepare oneself for bed. These satisfying or promoting routines make life easier and require less mental effort in regard to planning each activity. Some routines may be damaging. For example, Paul has an afternoon routine of leaving work, stopping at the local bar for a couple of drinks, and then picking up his children up from school. This pattern of behavior may be satisfying to him but also possibly damaging to the children.

While you are interviewing the client during the occupational profile process, you will find it helpful to ask the client about his or her daily routines. This gives you a chance to understand how certain occupations lead into others and the place each takes in the structure of the client's life.

Rituals

People perform *rituals*, or actions that have cultural, spiritual, or social meaning. These rituals are part of a person's identity, value system, and beliefs. Rituals often stem from cultural or social traditions or symbolic actions as parts of a belief system, such as a religion. For example, a family may have a ritual of having the smallest child place the star on the top of the Christmas tree (Figure 3-4). A couple may have a nightly ritual of praying together before going to sleep. Rituals contribute meaning to the lives of those who are part of the social or cultural group that values the events and actions that comprise the rituals. The way in which these rituals are performed will be unique to each client; thus it is important to understand their place in daily occupations.

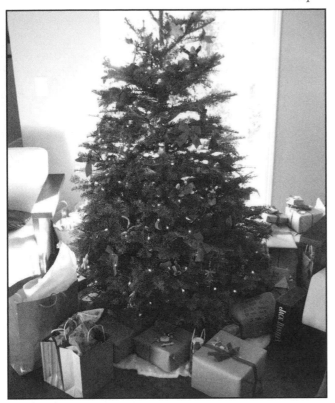

Figure 3-4. Putting up a Christmas tree every Christmas is a ritual.

Roles

The behaviors and actions expected of clients by their social and cultural contexts define the *roles* that clients encompass. A client can define and clarify what those roles are, as well as the occupations that each role entails. It is the social environment in which the client engages that sets the expectations for behavior in a particular role. For example, the role of a mother and the expected behaviors of mothers in some countries are very different from what they are in many urban areas of the United States. A client can identify with several roles within his or her life in many different contexts. For example, within the family Jennifer is mother, daughter, sister, and wife. At work, she is a public relations director, a confidante to her employer, and a coworker. As a member of her community, she is a member of her city council. In her social context, she is a friend. Understanding a client's roles helps to identify the occupations he or she is expected to engage in. It also gives perspective to the social demands on the client for the occupations that correspond to certain roles. For example, if your client is a mother of triplets, this gives you a deeper understanding of the occupations in which she must engage in her role of mother (Activity 3-8).

ACTIVITY 3-8

What different roles do you fill in your life?

CONCLUSION

Conducting an occupation-based activity analysis involves gaining an understanding of how the client defines his or her occupation and the multiple surrounding environments and contexts. The process of occupation-based analysis adds the components of evaluating the client's meaning and purpose for engaging in the occupation, as well as the performance patterns and the environment and contexts that support or hinder participation. All of this information can be gathered through the occupational profile interview at the initiation of services or as the therapy relationship expands. Through an occupation-based activity analysis, the clinician obtains a better understanding of how occupations can be used therapeutically and how open a client is to adaptations.

ACTIVITIES

1. Assess how each of your environments and contexts either supports or inhibits your performance in studying. Using Activity 3-9, give a brief description in each corresponding box as appropriate. If an environment or context neither inhibits nor supports performance, leave that box empty.

2. Over the next week, use the grid in Activity 3-10 to record each activity that you do throughout the day. Write down what you do each hour of every day. Do not go into too much detail but list a one- or two-word description for each hour.

3. At the end of the week, refer back to your list of roles. Using colored pencils or pens, indicate one color for each role. Go through the week of activities and highlight each activity according to the role to which that activity corresponds. You do not have to highlight each activity.

   a. Is most of your time dedicated to one role?

   b. Is there a role you wish you had more of on your schedule?

ACTIVITY 3-9

CONTEXT	SUPPORTS	INHIBITS
Physical		
Social		
Cultural		
Personal		
Temporal		
Virtual		

ACTIVITY 3-10

TIME	MONDAY	TUESDAY	WEDNESDAY	THURSDAY	FRIDAY	SATURDAY	SUNDAY
6 a.m.							
7 a.m.							
8 a.m.							
9 a.m.							
10 a.m.							
11 a.m.							
Noon							
1 p.m.							
2 p.m.							
3 p.m.							
4 p.m.							
5 p.m.							
6 p.m.							
7 p.m.							
8 p.m.							
9 p.m.							
10 p.m.							
11 p.m.							
Midnight							
After							

c. How would this look different if you were to suddenly become ill?

4. Choose an occupation that you find meaningful, and complete sections 1 to 4 of the Occupation-Based Activity Analysis Form found in Appendix B.

QUESTIONS

1. Why is it important to find out about a client's values and beliefs?

2. Using the example of washing one's hair in the shower, in what ways could an occupation-based activity analysis differ from an activity analysis?

3. What are examples of activities that can be spiritual but not religious?

4. In what ways can an occupational profile be obtained for a client who is unable to speak?

5. Your client Donny is an 82-year-old man who lives in a nursing home. He has a pet parrot and his primary goal is to be able to feed and give water to the parrot in his cage twice a day, as the nursing staff are not allowed to touch the cage. What are the physical, social, temporal, and cultural environments and contexts to be considered?

6. How are roles, routines, habits, and rituals different from each other? How might they be interrelated?

REFERENCES

American Occupational Therapy Association. (2014). Occupational therapy practice framework: Domain and process (3rd ed.). *American Journal of Occupational Therapy, 68*(Suppl. 1), S1-S48. Retrieved from http://dx.doi.org/10.5014/ajot.2014.682006

Christiansen, C. H. (1999). Defining lives: Occupation as identity: An essay on competence, coherence, and the creation of meaning, 1999 Eleanor Clarke Slagle lecture. *American Journal of Occupational Therapy, 53,* 547–558.

Crabtree, J. L. (1998). The end of occupational therapy. *American Journal of Occupational Therapy, 52,* 205–214.

De Vault, M. L. (1991). *Feeding the family. The social organization of caring as gendered work.* Chicago: University of Chicago Press.

Fiese, B. H. (2007). Routines and rituals: Opportunities for participation in family health. *OTJR: Occupation, Participation and Health, 27,* 41S-49S.

Hocking, C. (2001). The issue is: Implementing occupation-based assessment. *American Journal of Occupational Therapy, 55*(4), 463-469.

Miller, D. (1998). *A theory of shopping.* Cambridge, MA: Polity.

Segal, R. (1999). Doing for others: Occupations within families with children with special needs. *Journal of Occupational Science, 6,* 53-60.

Segal, R. (2004). Family routines and rituals: A context for occupational therapy interventions. *American Journal of Occupational Therapy, 58,* 499-508. Retrieved from http://dx.doi.org/10.5014/ajot.58.5.499

Wilcock, A. (1993). A theory of the human need for occupation. *Journal of Occupational Science: Australia, 1*(1), 17-24.

STEPS TO ACTIVITY ANALYSIS

Step 1: Determine What Is Being Analyzed
Chapter 2

⬇

Step 2: Determine the Relevance and Importance to the Client
Chapter 3

⬇

Step 3: Determine the Sequence and Timing
Chapter 4

⬇

Step 4: Determine Object, Space, and Social Demands
Chapter 5

⬇

Step 5: Determine Required Body Functions
Chapter 6

⬇

Step 6: Determine Required Body Structures
Chapter 7

⬇

Step 7: Determine Required Actions and Performance Skills
Chapter 8

4

Step 3: Determine the Sequence and Timing

OBJECTIVES

- Identify methods whereby to determine the sequence and timing of the steps of an activity.
- Determine the positive and negative aspects of each method for determining the steps of an activity.
- List the elements to be included when using procedural task analysis to list the steps of an activity.
- Understand how cooccupations can exist within occupations.
- Define how occupations can be nested within other occupations.

In order to understand an activity and the demands that activity would place on a person performing it, one must first clearly identify what the activity being analyzed is and then break that activity down into its component steps. Each step holds information that may be the key to successful performance. For example, if you were analyzing the activity of washing the hands, a key step would be using the soap. This requires reaching for the soap, grasping it (assuming that it is a bar of soap), bringing it to the other hand, and moving the bar over both hands. Looking at each of these steps adds a new action and challenge for the person performing the task. Being able to identify the steps and timing of an activity provides the foundation for a thorough analysis and allows for successful completion of the remaining steps. Without a clear understanding of the steps, sequence, and timing, the remaining aspects of the analysis will be incomplete.

ESSENTIAL STEPS

Determining which steps are essential to success in the activity or occupation will help you with this part of the activity analysis process. While each person may complete an activity differently than another person, it is important to understand which steps or timing elements are essential for successful performance of an activity. What defines *success* has been determined in the first step of the analysis process. Perhaps the activity is brushing the teeth. Success is defined by clean and healthy teeth. For common activities like this, there are clear ways to determine success. This helps in identifying the keys steps, without which one would

Thomas H
Occupation-Based Activity Analysis, Second Edition (pp 57-66).
© 2015 SLACK Incorporated.

not be able to progress through each step. An example of this is taking the cap off the toothpaste tube. This is essential in order to put toothpaste on the toothbrush. Without this step and completing it in the correct order, the step following this would not allow a person to brush his or her teeth. While in this example the essential step is easy to see, in many cases the essential steps may seem subjective or rely on what the client sees as successful completion. In the example of brushing the teeth, a client may not see the use of toothpaste as an essential step. This is where it is important to define the activity clearly. Brushing the teeth can be seen as a separate activity that is "nested" within the routine of grooming (we will talk more about nesting later in this chapter). So what defines grooming? The *Framework* nicely defines for us what grooming entails—obtaining and using supplies; removing body hair; applying and removing cosmetics; washing, drying, combing, styling, brushing, and trimming hair; caring for nails; caring for skin, ears, eyes, and nose; applying deodorant; cleaning mouth; brushing and flossing the teeth; removing, cleaning and reinserting dental orthotics and prosthetics (AOTA, 2014). However, what if we are analyzing an activity that is not defined in the *Framework*? What if a client defines success differently?

METHODS FOR DETERMINING KEY STEPS

Once the activity or occupation has been clearly defined, you must begin to list the key steps. Experience may allow you to mentally recall the steps of an activity that is familiar to you, but it is impossible to know the details of every imaginable occupation. For example, you may have a client who is hoping to return to his job as a pharmacist. Understanding the activities required of this profession, as well as the steps to each of the activities, can be done in several ways. There are pros and cons to each method for determining the steps required of an activity; however, the method we choose may have much to do with pragmatic factors such as cost and time.

Mentally Process the Steps

With simple, everyday tasks, the easiest way to determine the steps is to mentally visualize each step.

For example, if asked what the component steps are to washing your hands, you would probably be able to come up with the essential steps. However, with more complex activities, this may not be feasible. By simply relying on your own memory and understanding of an activity, many steps may be left out. The benefits of this method are that it takes very little time or expense. It is a technique that clinicians use continuously throughout the day, planning intervention sessions, conducting evaluations, and discharge planning with clients. Through experience, practice, and exposure to common occupations, the ability to mentally visualize steps evolves and the ease in which this occurs improves.

Engage in the Activity Yourself

While not always possible, engaging in the activity yourself gives you a perspective not possible with other methods. While the experience of an activity is different for each person, participating in an activity allows you to "feel" what it is like to participate in the activity and pick up on steps and elements that may not be detected through mental visualization or by watching others. There may be timing elements that are difficult to determine, such as the exact moment something should happen or the next step should occur. For example, if you were to write down the sequence and timing of flying a kite, you would probably be able to come up with the basic sequence (if you had ever engaged in this activity). But if I gave you a kite and asked you to set it into flight, you would find that there were many elements of timing that are not evident by just watching someone else do it or mentally visualizing it. To get the kite up into the air, you must use the airflow, which is felt through the kite string. By pulling on the kite string at the right time, the kite will glide up on air currents. Understanding this complex sequence and timing and the actions required is not easily "seen" but is felt. This is true of many occupations. It is often difficult to break down an occupation into a sequence of actions when the actions are not observable, or each step is reliant on external occurrences, or the outcome of a previous step.

Participating in an occupation or activity allows the clinician to gather a broader understanding of an activity, allowing for a more accurate analysis. It allows us to creatively find activities that meet our client's needs. If working with a client who has weak supinators, how might you find an activity that would require him to supinate his hand? As you sit reading this, are you supinating your hand, perhaps mimicking movements of activities? If you were to try to find an activity that requires this motion, you could begin trials of different things yourself. Does playing cards, brushing your teeth, folding paper, or using a phone challenge the supinators? (OK, try these.)

There are as many limitations to this method as there are benefits. Time is often the greatest limitation. Unfortunately, we do not always have the time to experience all of the occupations that our clients do (our employers are also hesitant to pay us to do so). Especially in the case of occupations that span great lengths of time, participating in them ourselves is not always possible. The contexts in which the occupations occur also limit our participation. For example, let's say we are analyzing the activity of ice climbing (Figure 4-1). The physical environment in which this occurs requires that we be in a climate that is cold (very cold) and have a surface covered in ice on which to climb. Ice climbing is typically done in pairs or with groups, in which there are social expectations of participation. Special equipment is also needed, such as spikes to clamp onto boots, a helmet, ropes, and other protective gear. There is also a certain amount of skill required, and body functions are needed to safely climb the ice and survive. The demands of this activity and many activities that our clients participate in limit our choice of the method whereby we can analyze the activity. Participating in the activity ourselves is limited not only by time and cost, but also by safety, our knowledge, the physical environment, and access to the tools and equipment.

Talk to Your Client

The person most intimately involved in an occupation is going to be your client. Asking your client to explain an activity step by step may give you an overall idea of how a task is done and the objects and equipment needed. The client may be able to give you information regarding aspects of the activity that cannot be seen by an observer. However, you must keep in mind that your client may leave out essential details, assuming that you already know about certain aspects of the activity or because he or she is unsure of how much detail to give you. Some clients may be unable to verbally give you the information needed due to cognitive or speech impairments. However, this is often the easiest and quickest way to gather information. When

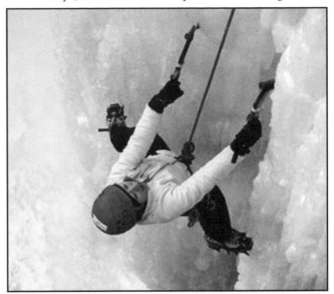

Figure 4-1. The activity demands of ice climbing are complex.

time and travel are delimiters, asking the client is often the most feasible option. When you are asking the client to give you information regarding an activity, it is important that you ask probing questions to gather all of the pertinent details. You will want to gather information regarding all aspects of the activity, including the objects and properties, space demands, and social demands (covered in the next chapter). For example, ask about the objects and properties, such as the size, shape, and weight of the objects used. If your client states that he or she uses a hammer, ask what type, how big, how heavy, and what shape the handle is. If the client states that he or she works in a garage, ask for a description of that space in regard not only to its size, but also the lighting, temperature, noise, and ventilation.

Talk to Someone Who Performs This Activity

When talking to the client is not feasible or does not give you enough information, talking to another person who performs that activity can often elicit valuable information. In the example of the client who is a pharmacist, gathering information from the client's coworkers or employer would be a valid strategy for finding out what activity demands are involved in his job. In utilizing this strategy, it is best to be prepared with a list of questions for the person you are talking to. Be ready to ask very pointed questions that allow you to gather all of the needed information at one time. Just as was the case with talking to your client, you may find that the person you talk with may not give much detail or leave key elements out of their description because he or she assumes that you already know certain details. Preface your conversation with a brief explanation of what you are looking for and the depth of your current understanding of the activities you will be discussing. Be respectful of the person's time and be prepared to be flexible as to the amount of time such people are able to give you. This is one of the limitations of this method—coordinating time between the clinician and the experienced person. It may be difficult to find someone willing to talk with you, especially in situations where the occupation or activity is uncommon (such as making prosthetic eyes); participants of the occupation are very busy (the mother of quadruplets) or the information is seen as private information (the activities of a monk from a certain sect).

You may find that there are cultural or language barriers to gathering the information. Those you attempt to talk to may not understand why you are asking or may be hesitant to share information with you. For example, several years ago, I had the privilege of working with a gentleman, a practicing monk, who had had a stroke. The garment he wore every day was an elaborate robe that wrapped around the body in different directions. One of the primary goals in OT was to teach him how to put on this robe by himself, despite the fact that he had the use of only one hand. Because of his physical and speech limitations due to the stroke, he was unable to show me how the material was to be wrapped. When a group of fellow monks from his monastery came to visit him in the hospital, I asked about the robe-wrapping process. The group of men looked offended and many of them looked away. I learned that they were not allowed to talk to women and that the process of donning the robe was sacred and private, not to be shared with others. Respectful of their beliefs, I had a male OT explain to them the reason for my asking, and one of the monks agreed to work with the OT on this task.

Watch Someone Perform the Activity

Watching your client or another person perform an activity can give you great information on the physical actions required, as well as the timing and sequence of steps. Through careful observation, the clinician can gather information regarding the strength, range of movements, coordination, and duration of movements required for a given activity. The clinician can also begin to get a sense of the mental, sensory, and speech functions required. This method works well in situations where the experience of the clinician is a limiting factor or the context of the activity does not lend itself to analysis in other ways. While observing your client participating in the activity may give you some information, you may need to observe another person participating in the activity if your client is not able to perform the activity completely or if you need more information than your client can provide. If you find another person performing the activity (in a similar context as your client's), ask the person if you can observe him or her. Explain the purpose for your observation and obtain permission to take notes. You may also choose to videotape the activity. This allows you to rewind and slowly analyze aspects of the activity at your own pace. Keep in mind that you may need to receive written permission from those you are videotaping, unless this is being done in a public forum. You may be able to find video information on the activity without having to record it yourself. In the example of the activity of ice climbing, you could observe others in two ways—in person or by video. Ice-climbing videos abound on the Internet and are available on DVD or video. This is a more cost- and time-effective method for analyzing the activity. However, the timing, sequencing, and actions used by another person may not always be the same as those used by your client. This should always be considered in conducting an occupation-based activity analysis.

PROCEDURAL TASK ANALYSIS: DETERMINING SEQUENCE AND TIMING

Yuen and D'Amico (1998) describe a technique called *procedural task analysis*, which is used by OT practitioners to help determine the sequence of steps for an activity. Their suggestions for this process provide excellent guidelines for determining the sequence and timing of an activity. While the *Framework* does not detail the process to determine the sequence and timing (Table 7 of the *Framework*), adopting a method that lends itself to a more accurate description of the essential steps leads to a precise analysis of the activity demands and greater ability to explain to or teach a client or caregiver. Thus, the suggestions of Yuen and D'Amico (1998) are used here as a guide for writing out the sequence and timing for an activity analysis.

Each step should include the following:

- An action verb
- How the action takes place
- Objects used or interacted with
- Time elements (if needed)
- Amounts used (if needed)

1. Determine what activity you will be analyzing. Be sure to break down larger occupations into smaller activities or tasks, so that the analysis will be much more feasible and understandable. For example, instead of analyzing the activity of skiing, you may choose to analyze one component, such as purchasing a lift ticket or getting on a ski lift.

2. Preparatory and cleanup tasks should be included in the steps only if absolutely necessary. Otherwise, these can be separate activities. For example, you may not want to list all of the steps required for getting prepared to play a board game; however, you might want to list the preparatory steps for a computer task (e.g., turning on the computer).

3. In writing out a step, be sure to begin the statement with an action verb. This verb describes what the person participating in the activity must do. These actions should be observable. Examples of action verbs are *grab*, *open*, *write*, and *step*.

4. The next part of a direction statement should include what the objects or environmental aspects are being acted upon. In the statement "squeeze the bottle," *squeeze* is the action verb and *bottle* is the object.

5. One of the most important aspects of the statement is *how* the action should be completed. This can be a simple word, such as *slowly*, or more descriptive words, such as *in the shape of a figure eight*. These descriptors can be placed at the beginning of the statement, at the end, or in both places. For example, "*Carefully* place the pieces of bread together with the *peanut butter and jelly sides going together.*" *Carefully* tells the reader that you cannot slam the two pieces of bread together, and the last half of the statement tells you how the pieces should be aligned.

6. Include time elements if the timing of certain steps or the length of an action is essential to the task. For example, if the activity were making cookies, you would specify when to take the cookies out of the oven. The directions would state, "Remove the

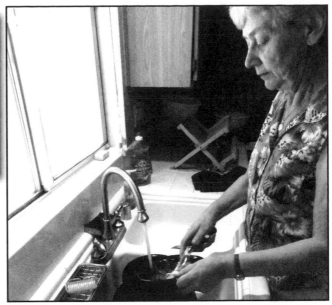

Figure 4-2. Washing dishes provides an example of how the steps must be separate: washing and rinsing.

cookies from oven using an oven mitt after 20 minutes." Often, the directions are not related to time but to other indicators, such as repetitions (e.g., "Stir pudding mix 25 times" or "Remove from refrigerator when pudding is a semisolid and no longer liquid").

7. List the steps in the correct sequence, as they normally occur. If a step or a sequence of steps recurs, state which steps to repeat and for how long (e.g., "Repeat steps 3 to 6 until all hair is removed").

8. Keep the steps simple and concise. Keep out unneeded details and avoid including multiple instructions in one step. A sign that you may be including too much information into one step is if there is the word *and* linking two action verbs in your directions. This does not always mean that you are giving two or more steps in one but is a sign that the direction may be too complex. For example, "Rinse the dishes and then put them in the dishwasher" is actually two different steps. The first half, "rinse the dishes," is the first step that needs further clarification as to how each dish is to be rinsed (and where). The next step would include putting the dish in the dishwasher. An example of where it would be acceptable to combine two actions would be: "Pick up the spatula and place it in the sink." This includes the word *and* and two actions: *pick up* and *place*. However, the actions link up into one simple step (Figure 4-2).

9. Be specific as to the amount of a certain material that is needed or used during a step. For example,

in describing washing the hair, you might state "Pour a quarter-sized amount of shampoo into the opposite hand." Use descriptors if exact amounts such as cups, inches, or numbers are not called for. "Enough to cover the page," "a pinch," "a handful," and "enough to fill the pot" are examples of describing the amount needed for a particular step. While the amount used for a step may seem intrinsically understood to you, for others it may be a novel concept.

10. One of the things he and I worked on was picking out his clothing for the day. I had to be very succinct and specific in the directions that I gave him, as he would often pull out four pairs of underwear, three shirts, and no pants. Until this becomes the new fashion statement of the day, I needed to be more specific about having him choose one of each type of clothing.

11. Some tasks are not as simple as following numbered steps that follow a logical sequence. There are times when the outcome of an action or an environmental situation has implications on the next action taken. This creates conditional statements (or "if/then" statements). If the task you are analyzing has many of these situations occur, or if the participant must make decisions that influence which step is next, you may choose to graph the steps in an algorithm. An algorithm is a visual diagram of the steps of a task based on information collected during the activity, and then specific options are given for the next step based on that information. Algorithms are used in professions such as mathematics and engineering to help with decision making and to standardize procedures. Health care has used algorithms to design protocols and clinical pathways (Miller, Ryan, & York, 2005). For complex situations, an algorithm can become very large and detailed, especially when there are multiple possible outcomes for each step. The idea behind an algorithm diagram is not to list the details of each step, but rather to help clarify the sequence of steps based on conditional aspects. See Figure 4-3 for an example of a simple algorithm for manicuring the nails.

12. Do not indicate to use the right or left hand unless absolutely necessary. This is also true for which lower extremity is to be used for a particular step.

13. Do not list the physical or mental requirement of the task. This part of the analysis comes later and is not included as part of the steps. Write out the steps as if you were going to use the list to instruct a client to do the task. You would not tell a client to "use vestibular functions to maintain upright position." A good way to check your directions is to read them aloud to someone, having them act upon each step. If it does not make sense, or the person is not able to act upon your direction, take another look at what you have included in the wording of the directions.

14. Include precautions and warnings for certain steps in parentheses. For example, a statement such as, "Do not touch the metal part of the iron to any body part" could be included in the directions for ironing. Some precautions can be included in part of a step, such as, "Wait 5 minutes or until the polish is dry before using your hands to touch objects."

15. Do not include proper nouns or specifics in regard to the objects and properties unless absolutely necessary. For example, you would not state, "Remove nail polish using Smith's heavy-duty polish remover and a cotton ball." In some instances, it is very important to include the name brand or type of material being used, as in recipes. A recipe for sugar-free cookies may call for the use of a specific sugar substitute. If a different sugar substitute were used, the amount used might be wrong and the end result might not be as successful.

16. While most activities can be completed in many different ways, Lin and Browder (1990) stated that in considering the steps of a task, clinicians must construct the steps in a logical order that considers "sociocultural norms," logical positioning of objects, safety, hygiene, and cost-effectiveness. This means that while you may be able to think of a variety of ways in which an activity could be done, you should stick to what is considered the social norm. This would be done only if you were conducting an activity analysis generically, rather than an occupation-based activity analysis. In conducting an activity analysis (not an occupation-based activity analysis), be careful not to create special circumstances or "could be" situations. In listing the steps of an activity, think of how the activity is typically done. As we progress through this book, you will see that completing an occupation-based activity analysis will allow you to include the complexities of different situations and ways of completing a task. For now, we are looking at activities in their simpler form as they are generally done by the majority of those who participate in the activity. For example, if asked to

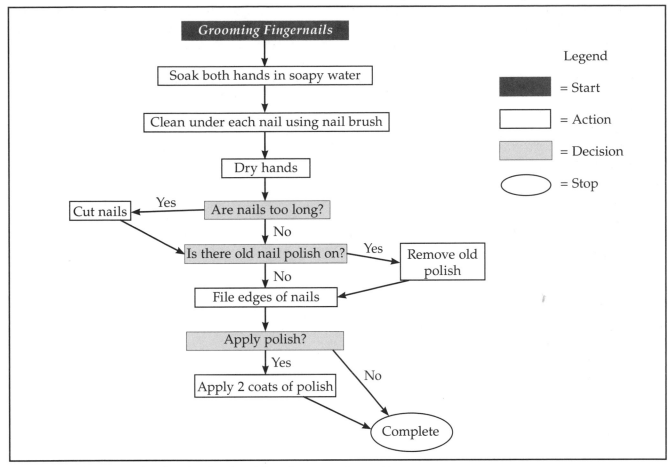

Figure 4-3. An example of a simple algorithm for grooming nails.

list the steps required of making scrambled eggs, you could describe an alternative method of making them in the microwave. However, this is not the typical method used, and thus the traditional use of a pan and stove should guide the analysis (Figure 4-4).

Complete Activity 4-1 to put these principles into practice.

CO-OCCUPATIONS

Many occupations and activities are not done alone and require engagement with others. Occupations that involve more than one person are called *co-occupations* (Zemke & Clark, 1996). This includes occupations in which social interaction is required or that rely on another person's actions. Caring for a child or a pet is an example of a co-occupation. For example, when David engages in leisure-time activities with his children, the activities in which they engage depend on what his children choose. After coming home from a long day at work, David may choose to relax and play with his children, which might include the occupation his children are engaged in, such as coloring (Figure 4-5). The fact that the steps and actions taken by the client rely on the actions of the others participating in the occupation makes analysis a complex and difficult task. In analyzing these occupations, keep in mind that the steps and actions required will vary and will need to be inclusive of potential actions by others.

A similar concept to consider is the idea of nested occupations, in which several occupations are conducted at the same time and co-occur. Nested occupations may be distinct occupations that occur together or separate occupations, such as listening to music and surfing the Internet. Analysis of these types of activities requires that each activity be looked at individually but that engaging in the other activities is recognized in the analysis.

The following is an example of how to write out the sequence and timing for making scrambled eggs.

1. Pick up the pan by grasping the handle of the pan with one hand and picking it up.
2. Grasp the can of nonstick spray with the other hand.
3. Hold the nozzle of the can at least 6 inches above the pan.
4. Press the nozzle down and spray the entire surface of the pan quickly.
5. Set the can of spray down gently on the countertop.
6. Place the pan on top of the burner.
7. Turn on the burner on by turning the knob slowly to the right until a clicking is heard.
8. Turn the knob slowly to the left until the flame is at a medium level.
9. Grasp one egg with one hand.
10. Tap the egg against the edge of the counter until a crack is formed.
11. Bring the egg above the bowl quickly.
12. Using both hands, place your thumbs into the crack and pull the shell apart gently, allowing egg to fall into bowl.
13. Place eggshell into the trash can.
14. Repeat steps 9 to 13 for the second egg.
15. Hold the edge of the bowl with the left hand gently.
16. Pick up the fork along its flat edge using your right hand.
17. Place fork into bowl and move fork quickly in circular motion.

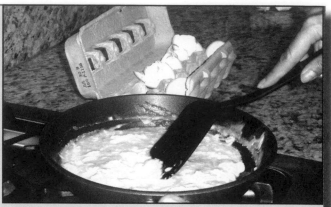

Figure 4-4. Making scrambled eggs.

18. Set fork down on countertop.
19. Pour the eggs into the pan carefully.
20. Grasp the handle of the pan with your left hand and pick up a spatula with right hand. (Yes, I combined these two steps.)
21. Holding onto the handle of the pan, stir the eggs slowly with the tip of the spatula.
22. Continue to stir until the eggs are fluffy and no longer watery.
23. Turn the knob of stove to the off position until the flame goes out.
24. Pick up the pan by grasping its handle and lifting it up carefully.
25. Pick up the spatula along its handle.
26. Tilt the pan over the plate and scrape the eggs out of pan using the spatula.
27. Set the pan down on the burner.
28. Set the spatula down on the countertop.

CONCLUSION

The process of breaking down an activity into its component parts is essential to understanding the complexity of an activity. It includes identifying those aspects of the activity you can see, such as actions, as well as those you can not, such as waiting for a specific period of time. It is important to identify those steps that are essential to successful participation and completion of the activity and the order in which they occur. There are many different methods by which to gather this information; some methods offer greater depth but require more time, while those that require less time and effort tend to lack accuracy. Each step of the activity should include an action, a description of how the action takes place, objects used or interacted with, and time elements (if needed). Describing the steps needed becomes more complex when others are involved, such as in co-occupations, where the actions of one person rely on the actions of another.

ACTIVITY 4-1

1. List out the steps required of washing your hands. Use the following checklist for each step:
   - Action verb
   - How the action takes place
   - Objects used or interacted with
   - Time elements (if needed)
   - Amounts used (if needed)
   - Precautions/warnings
   - No *right/left*
   - No *and* linking two action verbs
2. Now ask a classmate or friend to follow your directions as you read them step by step. They are not allowed to assume anything and must follow your directions exactly as written.
3. Write down which steps are missing or any missing elements. Are there hidden elements that you did not think of?

QUESTIONS

1. Why is it important to find out the steps required of an activity?
2. Fold a piece of paper in half lengthwise. On one half, write down all of the steps required of brushing teeth at the sink. Take those directions and read them to another person, having him or her follow each command exactly. Were there any steps missing? On the other half of the paper, have the person go step by step through brushing his or her teeth and write down the steps as you observe them. How are the steps you wrote down this time different than when you did it the first time?
3. List at least five things essential to determining the correct sequence and timing.
4. What are examples of co-occupations?
5. Describe a nested occupation in which you engage every day.

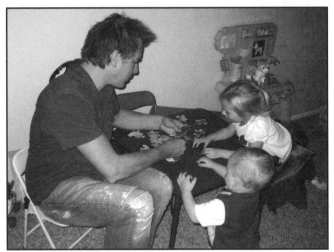

Figure 4-5. Co-occupation.

ACTIVITIES

1. Analyze the activity of shampooing your hair in the shower. Write out each step in the correct format, numbering each step. Analyze it as it is typically done, including all supplies in the shower.
2. You are working with a client who wants to return to the occupation of racing pine-box derby cars. Using your favorite Internet browser, find videos that will give you information on how this is done (also called pinewood derby racing). Write out the steps as described in this chapter.
3. Using the Occupation-Based Activity Analysis Form you started in Chapter 3, complete section 7 for the same occupation.

REFERENCES

American Occupational Therapy Association. (2014). Occupational therapy practice framework: Domain and process (3rd ed.). *American Journal of Occupational Therapy, 68*(Suppl. 1), S1-S48. Retrieved from http://dx.doi.org/10.5014/ajot.2014.682006

Lin, C., & Browder, D. M. (1990). An application of engineering principles of motion study for the development of task analyses. *Education and Training in Mental Retardation, 25,* 367-375.

Miller, T. W., Ryan, M., & York, C. (2005). Using algorithms and pathways of care in allied health practice. *Journal of Allied Health Sciences & Practice, 3*(2), 1-18.

Yuen, H. K., & D'Amico, M. (1998). Deriving directions through procedural task analysis. *Occupational Therapy in Health Care, 11,* 17-25.

Zemke, R., & Clark, F. (1996). *Occupational science: An evolving discipline.* Philadelphia, PA: F. A. Davis.

STEPS TO ACTIVITY ANALYSIS

Step 1: Determine What Is Being Analyzed
Chapter 2

↓

Step 2: Determine the Relevance and Importance to the Client
Chapter 3

↓

Step 3: Determine the Sequence and Timing
Chapter 4

↓

Step 4: Determine Object, Space, and Social Demands
Chapter 5

↓

Step 5: Determine Required Body Functions
Chapter 6

↓

Step 6: Determine Required Body Structures
Chapter 7

↓

Step 7: Determine Required Actions and Performance Skills
Chapter 8

5

Step 4: Determine Object, Space, and Social Demands

OBJECTIVES

- Explain how frames of reference and ecological models shape our understanding of the ways in which the environment can influence participation in occupations and activities.
- Understand how to determine the required equipment, tools, and supplies for an activity or occupation.
- Identify the properties of objects used during an activity and the influence these have on performance.
- Define the space demands of activity and their affect participation.
- Understand how to determine the social demands of an activity and how they affect participation.

Once the steps and sequence of an activity are understood, the clinician must gain an understanding of the objects used during the activity and the particular properties of these objects. Understanding the objects and space required allows for a greater understanding of the needed skills and body functions. For example, to fully understand the physical and cognitive demands of making a pinewood derby car, it is important to understand what supplies and tools are used in this process. Information regarding properties of the wood used (how soft or hard it is) and the types of glue and paint required will help clarify the needed strength, motor control, and other factors a person must have in order to make a derby car.

Understanding the objects that are required to perform an activity gives us another perspective on how the client will interact with his or her environment. Many physical and cognitive activities require that the person be doing something "with" a physical object. Try to imagine an occupation that does not involve objects. Even simple activities, such as walking or running, require objects such as shoes. By gaining an understanding of what is used to perform the activity, we can begin to look at what can be changed in order to allow for greater independence (covered in great detail in Chapter 9). For example, if we examine the occupation of self-feeding, the objects used include utensils, a table and chair, plate or bowl, cup, and, of course, food. If we are working with a client who has demonstrated difficulty with self-feeding, we will want to ensure that we look not only at what

Thomas H.
Occupation-Based Activity Analysis, Second Edition (pp 69-78).
© 2015 SLACK Incorporated.

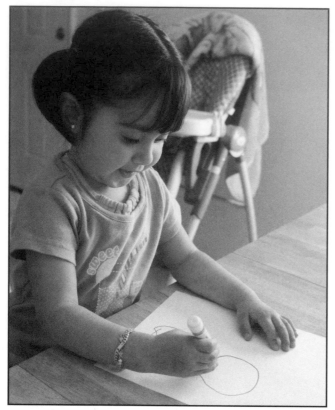

Figure 5-1. Tools and supplies.

are the objects with which we interact while we are involved in activities or occupations.

TOOLS

Tools used to perform an activity are objects such as scissors, pants, skis, or a stapler. While the most common image of a tool is one that might be used to do car repair or yard work, according to the *Cambridge Advanced Learner's Dictionary* (2009), a tool is defined as something that helps you complete an activity. Using a broader perspective on what a tool does and what it is used for allows us to think about how it applies to everyday occupations. What allows us to brush our teeth, comb our hair, or start our car every day? All of these are examples of occupations that require the use of tools. Tools are considered those objects that are not disposable and are reusable (they are not expendable, like supplies, which are discussed in the next section). In the example of brushing the teeth, the toothbrush would be considered the tool used, and the toothpaste a supply item.

SUPPLIES

Supplies are the physical articles needed to make or do something; they become depleted during the process of the activity. One definition of *supply* is that it is the substance or substances out of which things are made (*American Heritage Dictionary*, 2004). Supplies could also be considered substances that are consumed or expended during the course of an activity. For example, the supplies needed for writing a letter would be the paper (which becomes used the moment it is written on) and the writing utensil, which expends ink or lead—also a supply that cannot be reused (Figure 5-1). The *Occupational Therapy Practice Framework, 3rd Edition* (the *Framework*) lists paint, milk, and lipstick as examples of supplies (AOTA, 2014). It is important to recognize that supplies are objects that may need to be replenished at the end of an activity or after a certain amount of time (as in the example of paint, where the supply becomes diminished with each use). In identifying the supplies needed for an activity, it may be necessary to identify the amount needed (how much paint) and the properties of those supplies

is occurring within the person that could be causing difficulty (such as decreased hand strength or range of motion), but also at how we could change the objects used to allow for greater independence. Perhaps we could increase the size of the handles on the utensils to compensate for decreased hand strength.

In many of the models for OT practice—such as the Person-Environment-Occupational Performance model (Christiansen & Baum, 1997), Ecology of Human Performance model (Dunn, Brown, & McGuigan, 1994), and the Person-Environment-Occupation model (Law et al., 1996)—occupational performance is influenced by the interaction of elements within the person, the environment, and the occupation. Changes in any of these influence occupational performance. These models illustrate the need to thoroughly understand the occupation that the client is attempting to perform so that the demands of the occupation (such as the objects) can be identified as a possible focus of intervention. These models are called *ecological* models in that they address the relationship between the human (all physical, mental, and spiritual aspects) and the physical and social environment (Brown, 2009). Parts of the physical environment and objects (type of paint). Properties are discussed later in this chapter.

EQUIPMENT

In the case of activity analysis, *equipment* is defined as instruments or appliances that serve to equip someone to complete an activity (*Merriam-Webster Online Dictionary*, 2010). Equipment identified as required for an activity is often physically larger than the tools and may be a machine, such as a microwave oven or vacuum cleaner. Equipment can also be considered a set of objects that equip someone for a task, such as the hard hat, tool belt, kneepads, and gloves needed by a construction worker. The *Framework* uses a workbench, stove, and basketball hoop as examples of equipment. It is often a challenge to distinguish between tools and equipment. Tools are often manipulated or used by hand to assist in a task, while equipment tends to be larger or mechanical in nature. Technically, a piece of equipment can be used as a tool (an electric drill can be used to hang a picture). Whether you define an object as a tool or equipment is not essential; what is important is that you be able to identify all types of objects required of the activity, large, small, gas-powered, electric, or nonmotorized.

PROPERTIES

For many activities, the objects used must have certain inherent properties in order to allow for success in the activity. A *property* is an essential quality or distinctive trait of a physical object (*Merriam-Webster Online Dictionary*, 2010). The properties of an object are described in words such as *red*, *heavy*, or *industrial strength*. Often, a particular type of object is required, like a particular type of glue or paint. The properties of the objects used may be instrumental to how the activity is conducted, the time elements needed, and the skill set required. For example, *oil* describes the property of a particular type of paint, which has characteristics that demand very different actions, skills, and time elements than paint with a different property, such as *water paint*.

The properties of the objects needed for an activity as it is typically done are very different from those needed for an occupation in which a particular person participates. This is especially true of occupations involving a variety of supplies. For example, if you were to list the objects used to make a pine-wood derby car, the tools used to carve and create the car might differ depending on the builder.

To learn more about how the objects and properties of objects for an occupation can vary, I visited a derby car race held in Los Angeles. In my unofficial study of this occupation, I interviewed several of the racers and asked them about how they created their cars. Some of them had purchased a kit, which contained a preshaped car and some paint, and the builder used glue and other objects around the house to decorate the car. Others chose to start from scratch with a solid piece of wood and to carve out the shape themselves. Even with this method, the tools used varied in that the type of knife used was dependent on the builder's experience and preference. This is where naming the specific properties of the objects used is of great utility. Naming the properties is not only important for particular activities, such as cooking lobster (you need a large pot with a lid), but also for conducting an occupation-based activity analysis for a particular client. In the latter case, you will need to gain an understanding of the particulars of the equipment, tools, and supplies that the client prefers to use (Activity 5-1).

ACTIVITY 5-1

List all of the tools, supplies, and equipment used during the activity of making scrambled eggs:

- Materials:

_____

_____

- Tools:

_____

_____

- Equipment:

_____

_____

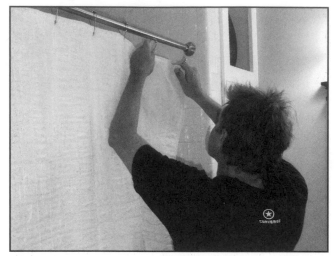

Figure 5-2. The arrangement of objects and the space in which an activity is conducted influences performance.

SPACE DEMANDS

Determining the space required for an activity calls for examining the type of physical environment typically needed in order to perform the activity. The type of environment can range from an indoor area to requiring a wall of ice running down a cliff. The area used to perform an activity may need to be at a particular climate with specific temperature, humidity, or ventilation requirements. For most activities, these elements have little influence on performance, but for others they are essential. For example, in painting the inside of a house, a certain amount of ventilation is required, the humidity cannot be too high or the paint will not dry, and it cannot be so cold that the paint will freeze. The demands for a certain temperature, ventilation, and humidity are strongly linked to the objects and their properties used in a particular activity. Certain objects may become unusable in certain environments (such as snow in a hot environment) or may become unsafe (like the fumes of glue in an unventilated room).

Size

The size of the area needed is the first aspect of space demands to determine. Analyzing the size demands for an activity requires the practitioner to consider what is absolutely required in order to perform the activity, not what is "ideal" to the practitioner. For example, if your client wants to race pinewood derby cars, how long is the track that the cars

are raced on? This will determine how much space is required to participate in this activity. There may also be demands for a specific arrangement of the objects in the environment, which will influence the size of the space needed.

Arrangement of Objects in Space

There are objects within the space in which the activity or occupation occurs. For some activities and occupations, those objects must be arranged in a specific way in order for the activity to occur. Certain objects may need to be spaced a certain distance apart or above and below each other. For example, in the game of chess, the chess pieces need to be arranged in a certain way before the game can start. When you take a shower, the soap and shampoo must be arranged so that they are within reach while you are in the shower. Thinking about the arrangement of objects for an activity helps us in planning treatment sessions as well. If we know that certain objects need to be placed in a certain position, we can arrange for this to ensure greater success for our clients. However, for many activities, there is no demand that objects be arranged in a specific way. Thus, in conducting an activity analysis, consider only the arrangement of objects within the space to the extent that this is absolutely required to perform the activity (Figure 5-2).

Surface

The surface required for an activity can range from a flat tabletop to rough pavement. As with all of the previous activity demands, the surface needed depends on the type of activity and the challenge you are seeking. Riding a bike can be done on many surfaces, but riding over rocks will be much more difficult than riding on smooth pavement. For some activities, the type of surface is not an option. Writing with a pen and paper, for example, must be done on a hard, smooth surface to be successful. In order to ski downhill, the surface must be smooth and at a slight incline. In racing pinewood derby cars, the same is true; the surface must be smooth, without obstruction, and at an incline. Thus, in determining the surface demands of the activity or occupation being analyzed, consider the slope, texture, and variation of the different surfaces being used during the activity (as there may be many surfaces required) (Figure 5-3).

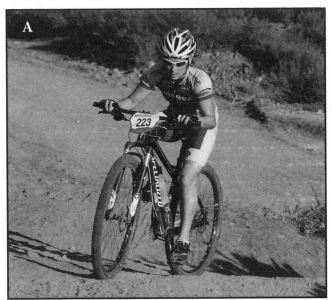

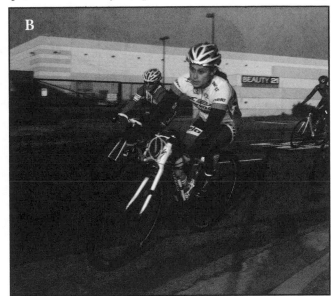

Figure 5-3. Riding a bike on (A) a dirt trail can be more challenging than on (B) a paved road.

Lighting

The next space demand to consider is how much lighting is required and what type. For some activities, the type and amount of lighting is not particularly important (e.g., watching television). However, when one is reading or conducting activities that require a high level of visual acuity, the amount and quality of light will be important. In considering whether lighting is important, ask yourself the following questions: Does the activity require visualizing fine details? Does the amount of light influence safety? Does lighting influence social interaction (as at a singles party)? Is lighting needed to establish a certain environment (as for quiet meditation)? The answers to these questions can start to uncover what lighting needs there may be for the activity you are analyzing. This is an area of the space demands that can be easily overlooked, possibly resulting in disaster. Several years ago, I planned a manicure group with several ladies who were patients at a hospital where I worked. I set up a round table and carefully laid out all of the supplies we would need. However, when the ladies began to work on their nails, I found that the lighting in the room was inadequate, and several of the ladies were not able to see well enough to get the fingernail polish onto their nails correctly. Focusing only on the supplies and surface needed, I missed a key aspect to this activity.

The light that is inherent to the activity should also be considered, as this will influence the skills and client factors required to participate in the activity. The amount of light may fluctuate throughout the activity, requiring the eyes to accommodate to the change from bright to low lighting (as in driving at night or through a tunnel during the day). The amount of light may depend on the nature of the activity, where there is either a low level of lighting (as in deepwater scuba diving) or very bright lighting (as in summer surfing). Of course, these levels of lighting are not required to complete the task but are a natural part of the activity.

Temperature

For most activities, having a certain temperature is not a requirement to complete the task. Having a comfortable temperature may be preferred by the patient or clinician, but it may not be required of the activity. So in determining the temperature requirements of the activity, think about what is absolutely necessary. For some activities, either heat or cold is needed, as with Bikram's yoga, which is done in a studio that has been heated to 105°F. This particular type of yoga is unique in that to be truly done successfully, the poses and movements must be done in extreme heat. Other activities, such as snow skiing, must be done in relatively cold weather, as the cold is what provides for the production and maintenance of the substance utilized to ski on: snow (Figure 5-4). It is often the objects utilized that determine the temperature required for an activity. Thus, in conducting an activity analysis, the objects and properties of the activity should be determined first.

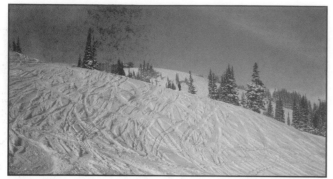

Figure 5-4. Space demands: temperature requirements of the environment.

In conducting an occupation-based activity analysis for a particular client, the temperature requirements may change, as you are determining what the temperature demands are for that particular person and in his or her contexts. For example, Pat has been an avid scuba diver her entire life. Over the last few years, she has been limited in her ability to perform many activities because of her rheumatoid arthritis. She is now able to scuba dive only in warm water. Diving in cold water causes disabling pain in her joints, and putting on and taking off a wet suit causes strain on the joints in her fingers. Pat now claims that she is only a warm-water scuba diver. If you were conducting an activity analysis on this occupation for Pat, in order for her to be successful at the occupation, temperature would need to be considered a requirement of the activity.

Humidity

Just as with temperature, a certain humidity level may be preferred by the client or clinician, but this may not always be a requirement. The objects and the properties of those objects utilized during the activity are often what determine humidity needs. For example, painting the exterior of a house requires a lower level of humidity in order to let the paint dry. The key to determining the level of humidity needed is to separate what is comfortable from what is essential. I am sure that those who live in areas of the world that experience very warm, humid summers would prefer to have lower humidity while conducting their everyday activities; however, this is not required for most people and activities. Just as the occupation-based activity analysis determined that Pat required a particular temperature to participate in her occupation, it can also determine a humidity requirement; the demands for a particular person in their contexts

may be different than the demands of the activity as it is typically done.

Noise

Noise, the type of noise, or the lack of noise is often a key factor to an activity. Imagine for a moment a high school prom with no music. The noise required for people to engage in this activity successfully is music played loud enough to facilitate dancing. In other situations, the lack of noise may be what is required. The activity of taking a test is an example of where the absence of sound is required for success in the activity. Typically, studying is an activity that one would expect to require quiet and minimal noise. However, if you conducted an occupation-based activity analysis with one of your classmates, you might find that he or she requires music in the background in order to study. Again, this shows how an occupation-based activity analysis may find different activity demands than those found in a standard activity analysis. In determining the noise requirements for a standard activity analysis, you will identify what the most common requirement for successful participation in the activity is.

The noise level that is inherent and produced by the activity should also be considered. Noises produced by equipment or people may not be required for success, but they are a necessary part of the activity. For example, the activity of vacuuming a rug includes the noise that the vacuum cleaner produces when running. In analyzing this activity, the amount of noise that is produced should be noted, as it may be a factor to consider in working with a client. For example, Hakima has a 14-year-old son, Neo, who has autism. He would like Neo to start taking on house chores, but the boy is hypersensitive to sounds and smells. In developing a list of chores with which Neo could help, you will want to analyze each as to the level of noise and smells they produce. Vacuuming would not be an activity that you would want to suggest for him.

The level of noise that an activity produces influences the level of tolerance to sounds required by the activity. An activity with a high level of noise requires a higher level of sensory processing ability. A lower level of noise may require a higher level of hearing ability. While taking a person's blood pressure, hearing a heartbeat through a stethoscope is required. The heartbeat is produced at a low volume level, demanding the participant to have a higher level of hearing ability.

It is important to also recognize and identify other elements of the activity that are instrumental to the demands of the activity and may impact performance. The environment in which the activity takes place or the objects utilized may generate sensations such as smell and touch. An odor may be emitted during part of the activity and may cue the participant to action (such as a burning smell when cooking) or may be part of the environment in which the activity is taking place, thus requiring the participant to be able to endure the scent (such as the smell of cow manure while milking a cow).

Other features of the environment or objects used during the activity may create sensations of pressure or light touch on the skin. Some activities may cause the skin to be wet (scuba diving) or have other moist textures touching the skin (applying shaving cream or lotion to the skin). The texture of the environment may be rough or considered "scratchy," as with building sand castles or walking barefoot in grass. In analyzing the environment and objects used in an activity, it is essential to identify possible sensory stimuli that may occur during the activity because in analyzing the activity for a client, his or her sensory-processing abilities will need to match the challenges presented during the activity (Activity 5-2).

Ventilation

According to the *Merriam-Webster Online Dictionary* (2010), *ventilation* is the circulation of air and the process of providing fresh air. In determining the amount of ventilation required of an activity, it will be important to understand the objects involved in the activity and the potential for emission of fumes, gasses, odors, and other elements that may become dangerous if inhaled. This is especially important when using chemicals, paint, or glue. Ventilation and the flow of air may be required to maintain a humidity level as well. The amount of ventilation required may also vary depending on the client and thus should be investigated in the occupation-based activity analysis.

SOCIAL DEMANDS

Social Environment

When an activity is engaged in with other people, in the presence of others or has an influence on others, social rules and expectations become part of the demands of an activity. Social rules are the typical norms and expectations of how one should act and communicate during the activity. Depending on the activity, there may be expectations of behavior toward other people participating in the activity, such as how one responds to a question or to another person's actions. For other activities, the behavior expected may not involve acting or communicating toward another person, but the actions or behaviors could influence another person. An example of this would be the social expectation that a person cooking food would wash her hands and not drop the food on the floor. For many everyday activities, there are unspoken social rules that are learned over time or as a child grows up.

Social demands are required in social environments, virtual environments, and cultural contexts. The social demands are often influenced by the culture in which the occupation takes place. Considering the social rules and demands in social environments

---

ACTIVITY 5-2

What are activities that typically require a high level of noise?

_____

_____

What are activities that typically produce a high level of noise?

_____

_____

What are activities that typically require a low level of noise?

_____

_____

What are activities that typically produce a low level of noise?

_____

_____

Other sensory features:

_____

_____

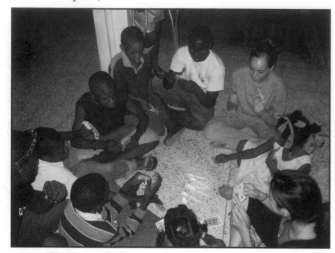

Figure 5-5. Social demands often include how participants are expected to interact with others, such as good sportsmanship or encouragement of others.

are what most of us might think of first and have been the focus of the examples given thus far. However, our engagement with others has expanded into the virtual world. Expectations for behavior have become the norm in certain virtual or online venues. How a person types, posts messages or pictures, and the timeliness of interactions are all examples of social rules that exist in the virtual environment. If a person were to post on the Internet or send an e-mail in which the text was in ALL CAPITALS, he or she would be seen as "yelling" online. On some websites, the use of profane language is discouraged, as are certain topics or pictures.

Social rules and expectations are shaped and determined by the culture and social environment in which the activity takes place. Therefore, in determining the social demands of an activity, the cultural environment in which the activity typically takes place must first be determined. For example, the behavior and social communication styles expected when one is eating in another country could be very different. In some cultures, it is rude to talk while eating, while in others talk is expected. Some cultures expect that women and children eat after the men, while in others everyone eats together (Figure 5-5).

In conducting an activity analysis of an activity as it is typically done, you will need to determine the social demands within the common culture of the activity. This may be difficult, as you will have to use your awareness of the activity, your observation skills of others performing the activity, and any written

information you may be able to find on the activity. In conducting an occupation-based activity analysis, consider asking the following questions:

1. Are there certain expectations of your behavior while participating in this activity?
2. Are there certain things that are not acceptable to others while participating in this activity?
3. Are there things you cannot do while participating in this activity because they might upset others?

Even activities that occur within the same country or culture can vary in their social demands depending on the social environment in which they occur. Some social circles have roles and certain expectations of behavior from the members of their society. For example, a teen who enjoys the activity of volleyball may have different social expectations when playing with his or her friends (such as yelling and laughing at each other, giving each other "high fives," and using words or terms not used with adults) than the social expectations when bowling with his or her parents. Understanding the different social contexts and various expectations will be important in conducting an occupation-based activity analysis. You will need to gain an awareness of your client's social roles and social contexts to help in determining the social demands of the activity. It is possible for a client to participate in the same activity but in several different contexts or social environments that make different social demands.

CONCLUSION

Gaining an understanding of the objects and environment utilized during an activity allows for greater perspective of the demands on the client's body functions and skill level. OT practitioners understand the relationship between the physical and social environment and participation in occupations. Just as with a challenging physical environment, the social demands of an activity can influence successful engagement in an occupation, such as the rules of a game or the expectations of others. The tools, equipment, and supplies also influence participation, as aspects such as size, shape, and complexity place demands on the client. Understanding how objects, space, and social demands play a role in an activity allows the clinician to develop strategies for adaptation and intervention.

ACTIVITY 5-3

Continue to analyze the activity of washing one's hair in the shower as it is typically done (not an occupation-based analysis on how you do it). Start by identifying which area of occupation it belongs to, as well as which subcategory, followed by the objects and properties needed, space, and social demands. Include the sequence of steps you completed as part of Chapter 3. See Appendix A for the full form.

1. Identify the activity or task:

AREA OF OCCUPATION (CHOOSE ONE):	SUBCATEGORY
ADL	
IADL	
Education	
Work	
Play	
Leisure	
Social participation	

2. Objects and their properties:

3. Space demands:

4. Social demands:

5. Sequence and timing:

ACTIVITIES

1. Continue to analyze the activity of washing hair in the shower by completing Activity 5-3.

2. Conduct an internet search on a common activity and find out how three different cultures vary in their social rules. An example would be riding a train.

3. Identify a common activity and list all of the variations in the tools, supplies, and equipment that could possibly be used. The variation could be in the properties of the objects.

4. Conduct an internet search to find out what the top five social rules are regarding e-mailing (or the use of a social media site). How do these influence how the activity is conducted?

5. Complete sections 5 and 6 of the Occupation-Based Activity Analysis Form you started in Chapter 3.

QUESTIONS

1. What is the difference between tools, supplies, and equipment? Why is it important to identify each of these?
2. List at least 5 examples of properties of objects.
3. What aspects of the space demands must be determined for an activity analysis?
4. In what situations would it be important to have a specific temperature or ventilation?
5. What are the social demands of traveling by airplane?

REFERENCES

American Heritage Dictionary of the English Language (4th ed.). (2004). Boston, MA: Houghton Mifflin Company.

American Occupational Therapy Association. (2014). Occupational therapy practice framework: Domain and process (3rd ed.). *American Journal of Occupational Therapy, 68*(Suppl. 1), S1-S48. Retrieved from http://dx.doi.org/10.5014/ajot.2014.682006

Brown, C. (2009). Ecological models in occupational therapy. In E. B. Crepeau, E. S. Cohn, & B. A. Boyt Schell (Eds.). *Willard & Spackman's occupational therapy* (11th ed., pp. 435-445). Philadelphia, PA: Lippincott Williams & Wilkins.

Cambridge Advanced Learner's Dictionary (3rd ed.). (2009). Cambridge, UK: Cambridge University Press.

Christiansen, C., & Baum, C. (Eds.). (1997). *Occupational therapy: Enabling function and well-being* (2nd ed.). Thorofare, NJ: SLACK Incorporated.

Dunn, W., Brown, C., & McGuigan, A. (1994). The ecology of human performance: A framework for considering the impact of context. *American Journal of Occupational Therapy, 48,* 595–607.

Law, M., Cooper, B., Strong, S., Stewart, D., Rigby, P., & Lettes, L. (1996). The person–environment–occupation model: A transactive approach to occupational performance. *Canadian Journal of Occupational Therapy, 63,* 9-23.

Merriam-Webster Online Dictionary. (2010). Merriam-Webster Online. Retrived from http://www.merriam-webster.com/dictionary/equipment

STEPS TO ACTIVITY ANALYSIS

Step 1: Determine What Is Being Analyzed
Chapter 2

**Step 2: Determine the Relevance
and Importance to the Client**
Chapter 3

Step 3: Determine the Sequence and Timing
Chapter 4

**Step 4: Determine Object, Space,
and Social Demands**
Chapter 5

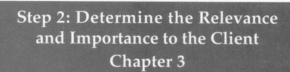

Step 5: Determine Required Body Functions
Chapter 6

Step 6: Determine Required Body Structures
Chapter 7

**Step 7: Determine Required Actions
and Performance Skills**
Chapter 8

6

Step 5: Determine Required Body Functions

OBJECTIVES

- Define body functions as they relate to client factors.
- Describe how to determine the extent to which a body function is challenged during an activity.
- Understand each of the mental function categories and how they are challenged and utilized during activities.
- Define each of the sensory functions and how they are challenged and utilized during activities.
- Understand each of the neuromusculoskeletal and movement-related functions and how they are utilized during performance of activities.
- Describe each of the cardiovascular, hematological, immunological, and respiratory system functions and how they are challenged during participation in activities.
- Identify each of the voice and speech functions and how they are challenged during participation in activities.

- Define each of the digestive, metabolic, and endocrine functions as they relate to the demands of participation in an activity.
- Understand each of the genitourinary and reproductive functions and how they are challenged during participation in activities.
- Describe skin and related structure functions as they relate to the demands of participation in an activity.

Understanding the demands that an activity makes for certain body functions requires taking a holistic look at all of the body systems and functions utilized to perform each step of the activity or occupation. It is for this reason that determining the sequence and timing of each of the steps first is so essential to a comprehensive activity analysis. The *Framework* utilizes the *International Classification of Functioning, Disability and Health* (ICF) to define *body functions* as "the physiological functions of body systems (including psychological functions)" (WHO, 2001, p. 10). Body functions are one part of the *client factors*, which include the values, beliefs, and spirituality, the body

Thomas H.
Occupation-Based Activity Analysis, Second Edition (pp 81-133).
© 2015 SLACK Incorporated.

functions, and the body structures that "reside within the client that influence the client's performance in occupations" (AOTA, 2014, p. S22). The body functions are listed in Table 2 of the *Framework*. According to the *Framework*, determining the demands of an activity during an activity analysis requires determining the extent to which each of the "physiological functions of the body systems (including psychological functions) (WHO, 2001, p. 10)... [is] required to support the actions used to perform the activity" (AOTA, 2014, p. S32) (see Table 7 of the *Framework*: Activity Demands).

Client factors are the features residing within the client that influence skill level but do not assure the skill level needed to be successful in an activity (AOTA, 2014). A person's physical and mental well-being affects his or her skill and patterns but is also affected by external aspects such as the demands of the activity and the context in which it is performed. For example, a person may have a certain level of vestibular and muscular strength, but that does not ensure that he or she will have the skill required to ski down an expert-level slope. Other demands of the activity influence successful performance in an occupation, such as the space demands (the level of incline of the ski slope) and the objects and properties used (the type of skis and boots used). As stated earlier, body functions and the other aspects of client factors can impact skill and success in an activity, especially if the body functions have been impaired by disease or illness. For example, a person with decreased muscle power will have difficulty maneuvering the skis around on the snow, and his or her skill level in this activity will be impaired.

An understanding of all of the steps required of the activity and what constitutes successful participation is needed to accurately identify all of the body functions demanded of the activity (and to what extent). All of the body function categories must be considered, as most activities challenge a variety of human factors. For example, in playing the game of tennis, not only are neuromusculoskeletal and movement-related functions used to run and hit the ball with a racket, but cardiovascular and respiratory systems are also challenged, as are mental and sensory functions, to see the ball and plan out a strategy to hit it. It is in determining the body factors required of an activity that the complexity of occupations is revealed. What might be considered a simple or everyday activity requires a complex combination of body functions, all working in conjunction.

In determining the body function demands of an activity, the occupational therapy (OT) practitioner must determine *to what extent* the presence or absence of a certain body function is required of the activity. In other words, how much is each body function challenged during the activity? The clinician must have an understanding of the physical, mental, and sensory challenges the activity poses for the human body. This is where the method used for gathering information regarding each step of the activity (as discussed in Chapter 4) becomes so important. If a clinician is analyzing an activity in which he or she is not familiar and the steps of the activity are merely mentally visualized, the clinician may not correctly identify the key body functions needed to allow for full participation in the activity. To begin to understand how body functions relate to the demands of an activity, this chapter asks the reader to analyze activities by rating the extent to which each body function is challenged. A body function that is not utilized during the activity would be considered not challenged at all, and thus on the activity analysis sheet, "none" would be marked. If *slightly* challenged, then the body function is utilized but very minimally. A body function that is utilized to a large extent is one that is challenged to a *great* degree.

There may be times when the extent to which a body function is required may be difficult to determine, as how much or how little a body is challenged is influenced by the contexts that surround it. Therefore, in conducting an activity analysis of how an activity is typically done, one must base the analysis on the context that is most common for that activity. Hypothetical situations or "what if" scenarios should not be considered in trying to determine what body functions are required. For example, if you were analyzing the activity of making scrambled eggs, you would not include the body function of divided attention because "maybe" the person has to also watch his or her children while making the scrambled eggs. Refrain from adding other elements within the context of the activity or adding other activities to the one you are analyzing. If you are conducting an occupation-based activity analysis, a full understanding of how the client typically conducts the activity as well as the contexts in which it is performed will need to be determined. The body functions required should be based on the list of steps you have already created in step 2 of the activity analysis, regardless of which type of analysis you are conducting. Using this as a guide will also eliminate the temptation to prematurely adapt the activity. For example, making scrambled eggs requires the use of both hands to crack each egg open. Yes, it can be adapted and done one-handed, but it is most commonly done with two hands.

ORGANIZATION OF THE BODY FUNCTION CATEGORIES

The *Framework* uses the ICF (WHO, 2001) classifications to organize the different body functions. There are eight broad categories:

1. Mental functions—Section 1
2. Sensory functions—Section 2
3. Neuromusculoskeletal and movement-related functions—Section 3
4. Muscle functions—Section 4
5. Movement functions—Section 5
6. Cardiovascular, hematological, immunological, and respiratory systems functions—Section 6
7. Voice and speech; digestive, metabolic, and endocrine systems; and genitourinary and reproductive systems functions—Section 7
8. Skin and related structures functions—Section 8

Within each of these broad categories, there are subcategories. The subcategories may delineate and help further define the different aspects of the broad category. For example, mental functions are divided into either specific or global mental functions. Under each of these subcategories lie specific functions, each with descriptions. For example, under specific mental functions, there are eight functions: *higher-level cognitive, attention, memory, perception, thought, sequencing complex movement, emotional*, and *experience of self and time*. Under each of these functions are common descriptors, such as *short-term, long-term*, and *working memory*—all for the specific mental function of *memory*. The body functions listed in the *Framework* are not intended to be an all-inclusive list, but are rather designed to be a guide for clinicians in understanding the underlying body functions that influence participation in occupations (AOTA, 2014).

SECTION 1: MENTAL FUNCTIONS

Specific Mental Functions

Higher-Level Cognitive Functions

Higher-level cognitive functions are described in the *Framework* as having the components of judgment, concept formation, metacognition, executive functions, praxis, cognitive flexibility, and insight. These higher-level cognitive functions allow us as humans to adapt to situations, think abstractly, and plan for the future. This category of functions is appropriately named higher-level in that the thought processes

SPECIFIC MENTAL FUNCTIONS	DESCRIPTORS
Higher-level cognitive	Judgment, concept formation, metacognition, executive functions, praxis, cognitive flexibility, insight
Attention	Sustained attention and concentration; selective, divided, and shifting attention
Memory	Short-term, working, and long-term memory
Perception	Discrimination of sensations: auditory, tactile, visual, olfactory, gustatory, vestibular, proprioceptive
Thought	Control and content of thought, awareness of reality, logical and coherent thought
Sequencing complex movement	Regulating the speed, response, quality, and time of motor production
Emotional	Regulation and range of emotion, appropriateness of emotions
Experience of self and time	Appropriateness and range of emotion, body image, self-concept

exercised within these functions are not basic but rather are complex in nature.

Judgment

Judgment requires mentally examining the aspects of different options and discriminating the variation in order to form an opinion or belief. We utilize judgment throughout our day, weighing options in order to make good decisions. Judgment is a difficult skill to learn but is closely linked to utilizing past experiences and knowledge in order to understand the implications of each situation or option. In order to form an opinion, one must speculate on the outcome and impact on not only themselves, but also on others. For example, if a person decides to answer his cell phone while watching a movie in a theater, this might be seen as poor judgment, as it has an impact on others sitting in the theater. However, if the person's wife is pregnant and is expecting the baby at any time, the person needs make a judgment call, which is a subjective decision based on the information available. This man must quickly weigh the implications on himself and on others if he (a) answers the phone or (b) does not answer the phone.

In analyzing whether judgment is required of an activity, ask yourself the following questions: Does the activity require the person to form an opinion? Is the person required to weigh options? Does the activity require that he or she understand the implications of each option? How much does this activity challenge his or her ability to make good judgments?

Real-world example: Mariem is 86 years old and lives in an assisted-living facility. Yesterday, she got a call from a "nice young man" who said that she had just won a drawing for a free trip to Hawaii. In order to process her prize, he needed her credit card number and social security number. Mariem found out the next day that her credit card had been charged to the limit and a new one opened up under her social security number. In reporting this to her credit card company, she admitted that this was poor judgment on her part. What information should Mariem have gathered before making the decision to give the caller her information? What else might have contributed to utilizing good judgment in this case?

Concept Formation

Concept formation is the ability to organize information and develop ideas based on the common qualities of objects or situations. Concept formation is linking pieces of information or sensory experiences to form an understanding of something that is not concrete. It requires being able to define how objects and ideas are different and understand how certain concepts or objects are related (Zoltan, 2007). Concept formation is closely tied to abstraction and generalization. Abstraction is mentally processing and coordinating ideas that are outside of concrete instances. Abstract thought is used to understand and apply theories and intangible concepts. For example, to understand the concept of love, one must link together notions of trust, caring, selflessness, and other nontangible concepts to create a concept of what love is and how this invisible feature of emotion and action evidences itself. Each person has a different concept of what love is based on his or her experiences.

To determine if concept formation is challenged during an activity, ask yourself the following questions: Does the activity require the person to mentally form concepts? Does the person need to mentally organize a variety of information to form theories or ideas? Does the activity require the person to understand abstract concepts (things that are not concrete)? Does the activity require that the person understand logical relationships between ideas (e.g., that roosters and dolphins are animals), yet also understand differences? Does the person need to understand opposites (e.g., small vs. large)?

Metacognition

Metacognition is having an awareness of one's own cognitive processes and the ability to manipulate and control one's own cognition (Zoltan, 2007). This self-awareness of one's cognitive ability is often defined as thinking about thinking (Brown, 1978). It is utilized to analyze a problem, monitor progress toward a solution, and plan strategies toward the problem (Flavell, 1979). Metacognition is important for effective learning, problem solving, and efficient communication with others (Al-Hilawani, 2003). Al-Hilawani (2003) measured metacognition by asking students to look at five pictures that each gave a different situation. The students were asked to sort out the pictures to find the one that did not fit the rest. While sorting through the pictures, the students were asked to verbalize how they were working through the problem. The researchers were examining the students' methods for obtaining and utilizing knowledge (Al-Hilawani, 2003). OT research and literature emphasizes the importance of metacognition for utilizing learning strategies—gaining an understanding of how one best learns and retains information (Munguba, Valdes, & Da Silva, 2008). Metacognition emphasizes the use of all of the other aspects of cognitive functions, such as judgment, memory, insight, awareness, recognition, and discrimination (Al-Hilawani, Easterbrooks, & Marchant, 2002).

Activities that call for metacognition are those that require learning new information (creating strategies for learning and retaining the information), as well as activities that require sorting and organizing information. In analyzing an activity for the level of metacognition required, ask yourself if the activity requires a person to have an understanding of his or her cognitive abilities. Does the activity require that the person analyze a problem and create strategies for how he or she is going to solve the problem? Must the person be able to monitor how those strategies are working?

Executive Functions

Executive functions are reliant on the frontal lobes of the brain and include complex goal-directed behaviors such as decision making, abstract thinking, planning and carrying out plans, mental flexibility, and deciding which actions are appropriate in certain circumstances (WHO, 2001). Many of the IADL activities we engage in every day require executive functions, as we must make accurate and safe decisions, think abstractly, and make and execute plans. An example of an activity requiring executive functioning would be planning a birthday party or a wedding.

Praxis

Praxis is the ability to carry out sequential movements, with correct timing and transitions between one movement and another. It is often called *motor planning*, as it relates to planning and executing functional movements. Humans develop praxis skills as infants, learning how to control movement, transitioning from a baby who is able to move randomly and nonpurposefully to being able to reach for objects or turn the head toward something of interest. Gaining praxis ability means that movements become more natural, in that we do not need to think about what we need to do in order to move (Figure 6-1). Think about when you brush your teeth in the morning. Do you think about how you are going to move your arm to reach for the toothbrush? Unless you are very sleepy, you do not have to think about it, and your arm automatically moves in a controlled fashion to reach forward and grasp the handle.

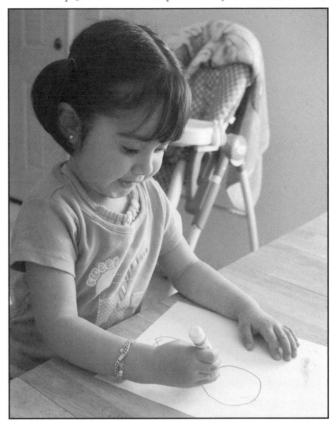

Figure 6-1. Writing requires a great deal of praxis.

Cognitive Flexibility

Having cognitive flexibility requires changing strategies in confronting a problem or changing a set of thoughts (WHO, 2001). This means that in being presented with two or more concepts, the person can shift from one to the other. When one is presented with new information, a new opinion or approach can be formed as needed for the situation. To get a better understanding of this, it might be easier to think of what it means to be cognitively inflexible. You may have met someone who was inflexible in their acceptance of a concept or idea despite how much you tried to inform him or her. People with little cognitive flexibility have difficulty changing strategies when there are changes in a situation or if there is an error (Parker, 1990). Therefore, in thinking about an activity and determining if cognitive flexibility is required, think about whether the activity requires the person to shift his or her thoughts as information is presented (Figure 6-2). Does the activity have the potential for error and require the person to change strategies? Does the activity require that the person shift from one idea to another?

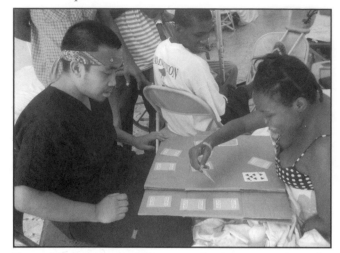

Figure 6-2. Cognitive flexibility: occupational therapy student using cardboard to create a table in Haiti.

Real-world example: Mary and John are out on their first date. They decide that they want to go to the movie to see the new romantic comedy that was just released and then have dinner afterward. When they arrive at the movie theater, they find out that all of the tickets for early evening show have been sold out. Only tickets for the 8:30 show are now available. Mary is terribly disappointed. However, John decides that they can go to dinner first and then go to the movie afterward. John's ability to change his plans based on the information presented demonstrates good cognitive flexibility.

Insight

According to the WHO's ICF and most OT literature, insight is related to self-awareness and having an understanding on one's strengths and weaknesses (WHO, 2001; Zoltan, 2007). This means having a realistic concept of one's physical and mental capabilities. Insight into one's abilities is required in order to make safe decisions and to correct errors when they are made. This is also essential to adapting to problems as they may arise or adapting to a disability (why use a walker when a person believes that he can walk just fine?). Insight is also closely linked to judgment, as having poor insight into one's abilities may lead to poor decision making and judgments. Insight is required for goal setting and in establishing future plans.

According to Barco, Grosson, Bolesta, Werts, and Stout (1991) and Crosson et al. (1989), there are three types of awareness that influence participation in activities: intellectual, emergent, and anticipatory.

Intellectual awareness is the ability to understand what abilities and weaknesses are present before engaging in the activity. With intellectual awareness, the person is able to verbalize any deficits that he or she may have. This is foundational for the other two types of awareness, in that without intellectual awareness, emergent and anticipatory awareness are limited. *Emergent awareness* occurs when the person is able to recognize limitations or strengths while they are occurring. *Anticipatory awareness* is the ability to predict or accept that a deficit will inhibit success or cause a problem (Barco et al., 1991). For example, a person may anticipate that he or she will not be able to climb the stairs leading up to the Lincoln Memorial based on an understanding of his or her abilities.

Awareness is necessary for activities that require advanced planning and the use of specific skills. In determining if awareness or insight is required of an activity, ask yourself if the activity requires having an understanding of one's strengths. Does it require that one be able to clearly understand what his or her weaknesses are? Does it require that he or she adapt tasks based on his or her weaknesses? Does the activity require setting personal goals? Does the activity require planning future events or achievements?

Real-world example: Dustin was out skiing with his buddies. At the end of the day, his buddies decided that they were going to ski the last run down an expert slope through a canyon. Dustin was not an expert skier, and he was very tired from a full day of skiing. Being aware of his current skiing ability, he decided not to join them on the last run and took an easier route down. This self-awareness and insight possibly saved Dustin from injury, as he might have hurt himself trying to go down a slope that did not match his skill level.

Attention

Sustained Attention and Concentration

Sustained attention requires maintaining concentration on one activity or stimulus for a sustained amount of time (WHO, 2001). Attention is focusing in on sensory information, choosing to process certain aspects of our environment or sensations. Thus, targeting our attention allows us to receive information, which also supports the retention of information in memory (Zoltan, 2007). Sustained attention requires vigilance toward maintaining thought and receiving sensory information. In determining if sustained attention is required of the activity you are analyzing, think about how long the person must sustain his or her focus on what is occurring. To what extent does the person have to focus? Are there opportunities for breaks or is continued focus required? An example of an activity that requires sustained attention is taking the National Board for Certification in Occupational Therapy (NBCOT) examination.

Selective Attention

Selective attention is focusing in on one or more stimuli, while all other stimuli or information in the environment are ignored (Zoltan, 2007). Selective attention requires actively discriminating between what information and stimulus to absorb and what to disregard. The demand for selective attention increases as the number of external stimuli increase. The greater the intensity of the distracter, the greater the demand for selective attention will be. For example, many husbands and wives feel that their spouses have selective attention when watching their favorite TV show or football game, as they tend to not hear when they are called. We may exercise selective attention in trying to study or read in a very noisy environment like an airport, where we need to filter out the noise and commotion around us to focus attention on what is being read. In deciding if selective attention is required of an activity, determine how many external distracters there typically are during the activity. Where does the activity typically take place? Does the activity require that the person ignore other stimuli while focusing on one stimulus or a certain group of stimuli?

Divided Attention

Divided attention is utilized when a person must focus on two or more stimuli at one time (WHO, 2001). Activities such as cooking utilize divided attention, in that while focusing on chopping vegetables, one might also be attending to a pot of boiling water. Parents often become experts at divided attention, as they are constantly watching what their children are doing while trying to complete other tasks around the home. Divided attention is what allows us to do several tasks at once (Zoltan, 2007). It may require us to divide attention between different motor movements, cognitive processes, or both. For example, talking on the phone and driving at the same time requires divided attention between two different sets of motor movements, cognitive processes, and sensory stimulation. In order to successfully do both, we must attend to both what we hear on the phone and say to the person, as well as what we see on the road and appropriately respond physically (turn the wheel or push the brake).

Shifting Attention

Much like divided attention, shifting attention allows us to engage in multiple tasks at one time. With *shifting attention*, we attend to one task at a time, but for limited amounts of time, refocusing our concentration on one stimulus and then shifting over to another (WHO, 2001). While divided attention requires that we focus on two or more stimuli at a time, shifting our attention provides attention to one stimulus at a time. For example, if a student is writing a paper, he or she might concentrate fully on typing the paper and then shift his or her attention to another stimulus, such as a cat or dog sitting nearby, and then back to the paper.

Memory

Memory is closely linked to other cognitive and sensory factors in that the brain stores information on sensory experiences (Zoltan, 2007). A person must attend to a sensory experience, such as looking at a flower, before it can be encoded into memory. If a person does not experience something by hearing it, seeing it, or feeling it, he or she will not be able to recall it from memory (e.g., one does not recall what a manatee is if he or she has never heard of or seen one). It is theorized that memories created out of sensations (sensory memory) are usually short-term and are stored according to the type of input (auditory, visual, or tactile). It is from this short-term memory that information continues on into working memory or long-term memory (Zoltan, 2007).

Short-Term Memory

The memory function that stores information temporarily, for about 30 seconds, is considered short-term memory. If not stored in long-term memory, this information is usually lost (WHO, 2001). Short-term memory is very limited and differs from working memory. It is what allows us to recall small chunks or bits of information for immediate use. For example, if you were to look up a phone number, you might look at the phone number (or parts of it) and temporarily store it in your short-term memory long enough to dial the number on your phone. In determining if short-term memory is required of an activity, you will first need to determine if it is working memory or short-term memory that is needed. Short-term memory is used for small pieces of information that are required only briefly. It may be used to allow a person to move on to the next step of an activity (did I look both ways before crossing the street?). It is possible for an activity to require short-term memory as well as working memory.

Working Memory

Working memory retains information while we are using it during a task (Levy, 2005). It is also believed that temporary memory allows for manipulation of information (Zoltan, 2007). It is working memory that allows us to hold information and use it during tasks. It is theorized that our working memory can handle seven pieces of information at one time (Parente & Anderson, 1991). We utilize working memory throughout our daily activities, such as in writing a letter, manipulating information, and retrieving memories to write each sentence that links to the paragraph and to the paragraphs that make up a letter. In this example, the person writing the letter can go back and read what he or she has already written, which would be an inefficient way of completing the task. It is working memory that allows us to problem solve and process tasks that do not involve physical cues to the information (Zoltan, 2007). For example, when asked a question in class, students may utilize working memory to think through the question and store information regarding other students' answers in order to come up with their own answer. It is working memory that allows us to perform many of our everyday tasks that require a temporary grasp of information for use in various aspects of the activity. Working memory might be used in order to create a strategy in a game by recalling an opponent's moves and actions.

In determining if working memory is required of an activity, look through the steps required and decide if any of these steps require mental manipulation of different pieces of information (you will actually be using working memory to do this). Does the activity require the person to recall and utilize chunks of information temporarily? (These are not intended to be long-term memories.) Does the activity require one to utilize memories to guide actions? Does the activity require complex problem solving?

Long-Term Memory

Information about past events, language, and sensory experiences that are stored for long periods of time is part of the long-term memory system (WHO,

2001). These memories are retained from a few hours to many years (Zoltan, 2007). This allows for the utilization of past experiences in order to deal with current ones. Information that is used during working memory is retained and encoded into long-term memory. Thus, information that is rehearsed or utilized as working memory is more efficiently stored long-term (Zemke, 1994). An example of long-term memory is recalling how to ride a bike, even after years of not having done so. We utilize long-term memory for activities that are repeated on a daily basis, such as brushing our teeth and driving home. Long-term memories are used for activities that require the ability to recall personal information (such as birth date and social security number), events (such as where you were yesterday at noon), facts (such as who the president is), and procedures (such as how to complete a task). When determining if an activity requires long-term memory, think about how far back they must remember. Do they need to remember events or information from over an hour ago? Do they need to recall how to do something they had done in the past? Do they need to be able to recall personal history?

Real-world example: Judi was attending a workshop where the speaker was using a VHS tape for her presentation. During the presentation, the tape became entangled in the player, causing it to break. The speaker was in a panic. Judi helped the speaker remove the tape and, to the speaker's surprise, she was able to restore it. Judi's first job while in high school had been working at a video rental store. Thus, Judi was able to remember how to repair a VHS tape, as she had repeatedly done at the rental store. The result was also a surprise to Judi, as this was not a skill she ever expected to use again; she was pleased to see that her repair job allowed the speaker to continue her presentation.

Perception

Discrimination of Sensations: Auditory

Auditory perception allows for the ability to discriminate between different sounds, tones, and pitches (WHO, 2001). This is what allows us to differentiate between the sound of a refrigerator running and rain hitting the pavement outside. Perception of sound is different from the ability of the ear to transmit sound to the brain. Perception of sound relies on the brain to interpret signals sent from the ear about auditory information occurring in the environment. It is what allows us to understand an alerting noise (a scream) from a loud radio. This is not to be confused with auditory memory, which is the ability to remember what certain environmental stimuli sound like (such as remembering the sound of a good friend's voice). Auditory perception is utilized for tasks that require a person to distinguish between two or more different noises. It is required when the activity requires the person to take action based on a certain sound (such as with a fire alarm or ringing phone). Discrimination of different tones and pitches is used in communicating, singing, or playing musical instruments. Being able to discriminate between tones, pitches, and types of sounds is essential for interpreting much of what occurs in the environment (e.g., watch a movie on mute and see how much is missed or can be misunderstood). Different tones may help in determining where an activity is occurring or how. For example, a mother may listen outside the doorway of the bathroom where her child is supposed to be bathing, listening for specific sounds that tell her that the child has actually entered the bathtub and is washing.

In determining if discrimination of auditory information is required of an activity, think about what actions are demanded of the person during the activity, not what ambient noise occurs during the activity. If discrimination of auditory information is required, the person engaged in the activity will be required to react or make decisions based on the sounds made in the environment. Does the ability to discriminate between sounds contribute to the person's ability to engage in the activity or can it be done without? For example, attending a musical concert requires this function, while taking a shower does not. Both include noise, but taking a shower does not require the person to utilize the ability to discriminate or understand the noise made during the activity.

Discrimination of Sensations: Tactile

Tactile discrimination allows us to distinguish different textures by touch (WHO, 2001). It is our ability to perceive the difference in textures, not just the body's ability to sense touch (which is addressed further on). Tactile discrimination is a perceptual function that gives us the ability to understand dimensions and physical characteristics of objects and determine if something is smooth or rough by touching it with some part of our body. Notice that this is under the category of "specific mental functions" because this function relies on the brain to interpret what is being felt.

Because we have a greater number of touch receptors in our fingers, humans tend to use their hands

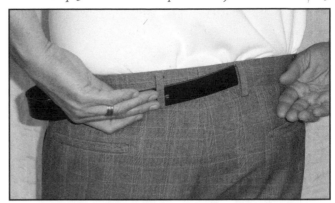

Figure 6-3. Using tactile discrimination to thread a belt through loops on pants.

to "feel" or touch objects (Cooper & Abrams, 2006). Thus, when we use our hands (or feet) to complete tasks, we may be using our sense of touch to give us information about performance. This is especially true when aspects of the activity are conducted out of sight or information cannot be gathered through sight alone. For example, in stringing a belt through the belt loops of a pair of pants, a person must feel for the loops with his or her fingers and use the sense of touch to feel for the belt in order to pull it through (Figure 6-3). If the pants, the loops, and the belt all felt the same, the task would be very difficult to complete. Think about what allows you to put your hands in your purse of backpack and find an object without looking. Tactile discrimination is what allows us to process what we are feeling and understand the difference between two very similar objects, such as a pen and a pencil.

Tactile discrimination is required of an activity if the person engaging in the activity must discriminate between different textures, such as smooth or rough, oily or dry, and sticky or smooth. It may also be required if aspects of the activity are done without the use of sight. Think about some of the daily activities you do that use your sense of touch: shampooing your hair (feel if there are soap suds left), typing (feeling for the keys), buttoning buttons, or turning pages of a book.

Discrimination of Sensations: Visual

Visual discrimination is our ability to perceive and interpret visual information. It is what allows us to discriminate between different shapes, objects, and colors (WHO, 2001). It is important to distinguish the difference between visual discrimination as a perceptual function and vision as a sensory function. *Visual perception* is the cognitive processing of what our eyes

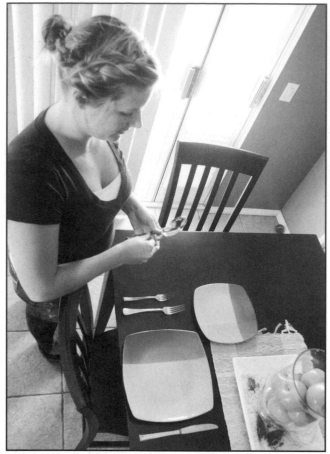

Figure 6-4. Setting the table is an example of the use of visual discrimination skills to discern the differences between the silverware and where to place the different items

detect. A person may have perfect oculomotor skill and intact eye structures, yet be unable to perceive or understand what he or she sees. Often referred to as *form discrimination* in the literature on visual perception, visual discrimination is primarily utilized to distinguish shape but also serves to distinguish and identify color, orientation, and edge (Zoltan, 2007). This is what allows us to react to the environment and interact with objects and people. Visual perception is required for a large majority of our everyday activities and works in conjunction with many other body functions for basic tasks such as standing or sitting upright or reaching for an object (Zoltan, 2007). To give you an example of how this function is used, set this book down, get up, and go to the bathroom (yes, even if you don't have to go). As you travel, think about how you understand what you are seeing and what allows you to take the correct path and use the correct objects.

Are you back? To complete this activity, you used your visual discrimination skills to set your book down on a solid surface (it is this function that tells

you where to place a book so it is not hanging off the edge of a table), to get up and walk toward a doorway or hallway and center your body as to not hit anything, to identify which is a bathroom, to place your hands on the door and push or pull as you see is needed, and finally to visually identify how to walk in. How did you know which object was the toilet? How did you tell the difference between the toilet paper and a towel? (Hopefully you chose the correct one.) So much of what we do every day utilizes this ability to discriminate between objects, shapes, and colors (Figure 6-4).

Discrimination of Sensations: Olfactory

The use of olfactory discrimination is what allows for distinguishing differences in smells (WHO, 2001). It is what might alert us to a smell that requires action, such as smoke or fumes. It may be used to enable us to tell whether something is rotten (as by smelling a carton of milk after its expiration date to determine whether it is still good). Many parents use olfactory discrimination to determine if their child needs a diaper changed or if their teenage son needs to take a shower. There are many activities that involve the presence of smells, but in determining if olfactory discrimination is required, you must determine if participation in the activity requires that the person engaging in the activity must use this function in order to perform that activity. Does the activity require that the person act upon certain smells? Does the person need to be able to detect the absence or presence of certain aspects, such as whether there are fumes from paint or glue in the air so that ventilation is needed?

Discrimination of Sensations: Gustatory

Our ability to discriminate between tastes is what allows us to determine sweet, salty, spicy, sour, or bitter. As a mental function, this is our brain's ability to discriminate between these sensations based on input from our taste buds. We must discriminate between certain tastes when we are preparing a meal or determining whether something we are eating is too salty or perhaps has gone bad.

Discrimination of Sensations: Vestibular

Vestibular perception allows you to determine the position of your body in space. This is what allows you to determine how to hold yourself upright or in a certain position for an activity (de Bruin, 2008). Perception of vestibular input is what tells you in what

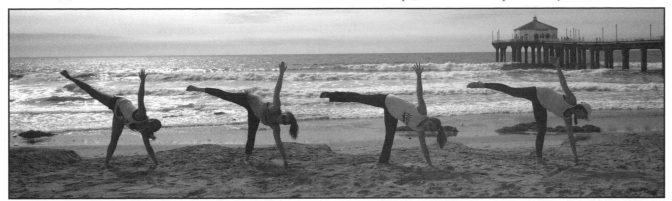

Figure 6-5. Yoga poses often challenge the vestibular system.

direction you are moving, the speed of your movement, your head position, and the position of your body in space (WHO, 2001). This requires mentally processing the positional signals sent from the inner ear that indicate the position of the head.

To determine if this function is required of an activity, think about what positions or positional changes occur during the activity. Does the activity require that the participant bend over and then come to an upright position again? Does he or she need to be able to position his or her body in a certain direction? Does the position of his or her head change during the activity? Is vision occluded or limited, so that the person must take a position based on vestibular sense instead of by sight? An example of this is dancing, where body parts are moving outside of sight, the position of the head may rotate, and the dance may require leaning to one side and bending down but then coming back to an upright position. This perceptual ability contributes greatly to balance as well (Figure 6-5).

Discrimination of Sensations: Proprioceptive

Proprioception is detecting muscle lengthening and shortening and how fast and in which direction a limb or body part is moving. The combination of vestibular and proprioceptive perception allows you to understand where your head and body parts are in relation to one another. This body function entails the interaction of the two to create a perception of where your body is in space (Figure 6-6).

To determine if this function is required of an activity, think about what positions or positional changes occur during the activity. Does the activity require that the participant move the body in a certain way without using sight to guide these movements? Does the activity require that the person understand and regulate how quickly his or her body is moving? Is

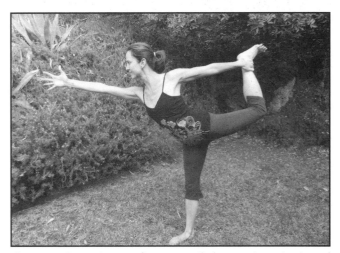

Figure 6-6. Discrimination of senses: vestibular-proprioception is used in great amounts in yoga.

vision occluded or limited and thus the person must take positions based on proprioceptive sense instead of on sight? An example of this is tennis, where body parts are moving outside of sight, the positions of the limbs are unequal, and movements are outside of the participant's vision (Figure 6-7).

Thought

Control and Content of Thought

Maintaining a stream of thoughts that relate to the activity or issue is appropriate thought content. In writing out a shopping list, we would be thinking about what is needed in regard to food and materials within the home. Thinking about the appropriate things during an activity sounds much like attention, but it is different in that this is related to the content of thoughts, not the ability to focus. For example, during a lecture in class, you might be utilizing attention functions to attend to the speaker but also your

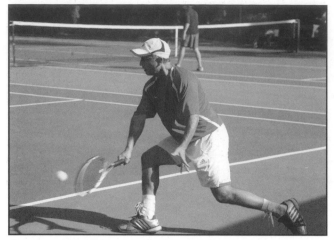

Figure 6-7. When playing tennis, the player relies on proprioceptive sense to know where he is holding the tennis racquet.

thought functions to think about the topic being discussed. If the speaker is discussing OT intervention for someone who has had a cerebrovascular accident and you are thinking about spinal cord injuries, you are not thinking appropriately. This comes under the category of "thought functions" for a reason; it requires mentally utilizing information that relates to the concept or activity at hand.

In determining whether logical thought content is required of an activity, think about what actions are required of the person—does the person need to act in an appropriate way (especially important when interacting with others)? Does the activity require that he or she think about aspects that all relate to the particular topic, such that the ideas or conceptualization utilizes information that is appropriate to the situation? For example, if you were designing a tree house, you would have to think about the appropriate tools and designs, who will be climbing into the tree house, and what it will be used for. Going over these concepts is important and appropriate for the task at hand. A person doing this would not be thinking about other things, such as what hair color looks best on Nicole Kidman.

Awareness of Reality

Distinguishing between thoughts and what is truly occurring requires an awareness of reality. This is how we determine what is real and what is fiction or what we are simply envisioning in our minds. A person who has difficulties with awareness of reality might believe

that what he or she sees occurring in a television show is actually occurring. Awareness of reality is what allows us to understand what is real in our existence (e.g., knowing that we cannot fly merely by donning a cape). With this also comes an understanding of what is feasible given the context and separating what might be envisioned in the mind from what is going on in reality. This requires separating dreams, imagination, delusions, or hallucinations from what is occurring in the actual environment.

To determine if this factor is required, think about how much the person is interacting with the environment and others during the activity. Does it require that he or she be able to distinguish between what is real and what is not? Does the activity demand that the person understand what is feasible and realistic given the constraints of the environment (such as understanding that one cannot make snowballs in the middle of summer)?

Logical and Coherent Thought

For thought processes to be logical and coherent, they must be reasonable and capable of being explained in words or symbols and used for reasoning. Logical reasoning requires using factual information and understanding how it relates to a problem or situation (Barnard, 1995). Logical thought is what allows our actions to be feasible; we utilize what we know to make decisions that "make sense." Sound reasoning requires this ability to think logically, which is needed for many activities that call for precise planning and understanding of facts or concepts. This might also be seen as common sense or thinking through a concept using available information. Often, the speed at which an action must be taken determines if logical or coherent thought would be used. Think about a time you were surprised, caught off-guard, or were in an emergency situation. Did you react logically or in a reactive way? One of my roommates in college ran down three flights of stairs during an earthquake and did not realize what she was doing until she was at the bottom of the stairs and the earthquake was over. This course of action was not logical; if given time to think about it, she might have acted differently. Many of our everyday activities require logical thought, such as balancing a checkbook, shopping for groceries, driving, and choosing what clothes to wear (Figure 6-8).

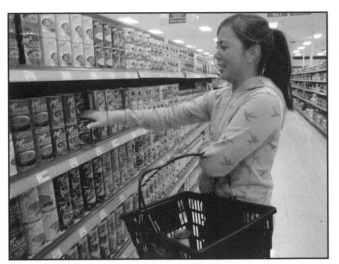

Figure 6-8. Shoppers must use logical and coherent thought processes while grocery shopping.

Sequencing Complex Movement

Regulating the Speed, Response, Quality, and Time of Motor Production

Executing movement patterns, as a cognitive function, is the process of mentally sequencing and coordinating purposeful movements (WHO, 2001). This includes the mental planning of how quickly we move, the timing of our movements, and limited extraneous movements (such as toe tapping or hand wringing). When you reach out to pick up a book, it requires not only the strength within your upper extremity, but also the mental ability to send the message from your brain to your arm how to move to actually pick up the book. Without this, your arm might flail about aimlessly or not move at all. This function is not related to physical ability or skill; it is the mental aspect of planning movements. It is separate from understanding what movements are needed, such as thinking about reaching forward to pick up book; it is the mental control over the movements as they are occurring (the execution).

The function of mentally sequencing complex movement is utilized when any purposeful movement is conducted during an activity. Therefore, almost all activities that require physical movement will require sequencing of movement. We learn how to sequence complex movements over time; as we grow and develop as children, we learn how to control our movements in purposeful ways, as well as how to move in certain situations (Figure 6-9). For example, the sequencing of movements required for snow skiing is not inherently understood but is learned over time and instruction. Thus, during the activity of skiing, the person

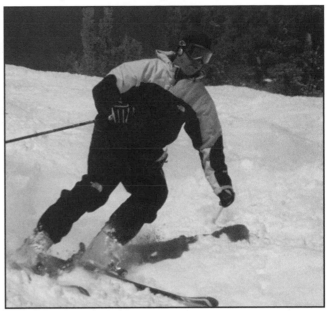

Figure 6-9. Righting and supporting can be challenged when the environment changes the position of the body.

engaging in this activity will need to rely on this factor to correctly activate the appropriate muscles and move his or her limbs and trunk in the sequence that he or she has learned to safely ski down a hill. So many of our everyday activities require sequencing of motor movements. Think about how much you have done today: showered, got dressed, brushed teeth, styled hair—all of these required sequencing of movements to varying degrees. When determining the extent to which this factor is challenged for an activity, think about how complex the movements are. Are the movements required part of a learned task or activity (much like skiing) and intrinsic to normal development (like picking up a book)? Is there timing of movements required or quick responses? Does the activity require that the person control extraneous movements such as tapping, hand wringing, or flapping (Figure 6-10)?

Emotional

Regulation and Range of Emotion

The specific mental functions related to emotions include feeling and demonstrating the affective components of the processes of the mind (WHO, 2001). This includes feeling and demonstrating sadness, happiness, love, fear, anger, hate, tension, anxiety, joy, and sorrow. In activity analysis, determining the requirements of emotion is very much linked to the social demands of the activity (see Chapter 5). The range and regulation of emotion required of an activity would be

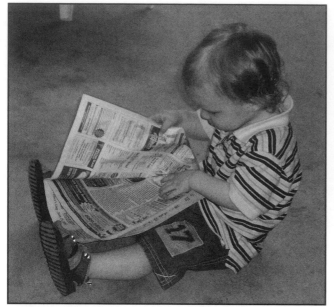

Figure 6-10. Turning the pages of a newspaper requires regulating the speed and quality of movements.

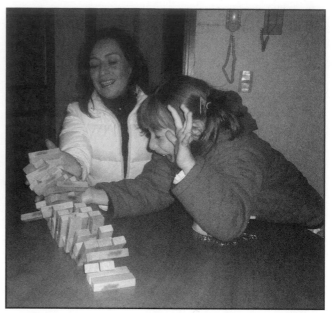

Figure 6-11. Playing a game often challenges the players to regulate their emotions when things do not go their way.

more linked to the affective aspects (what emotions are demonstrated) vs. those just felt. For example, in opening a gift from a friend, from an activity analysis perspective, the emotions felt are not required as much as the emotions that are demonstrated. Demonstrating a range of emotion is linked to successfully engaging in social activities.

While demonstrating emotions is important for social activities, feeling and regulating emotions is important when handling a crisis or decisive turning points in life or situations (WHO, 2001). How actions are carried out or decisions are made during difficult times all involve regulating emotions. This is also utilized during times of danger or following a catastrophe. Activities that challenge our ability to regulate emotions are those that surround specific contexts or situations. It is often used when a response to a traumatic or negative event is required. For example, a child participating in a spelling bee is going to need to regulate her emotions, as she may not win or may be faced with embarrassing failures.

In determining if regulating emotions is required of an activity, you must first determine what difficulties or possible dangers are most commonly encountered as part of this activity. Take precaution to not fabricate "what if" situations for common activities (such as riding a bike by thinking about what if one were to be hit by a bus). Think of only situations that are most common and likely for that activity. For example, skiing requires very little coping as most of the time the

most danger that will require any action would be a large fall. The activity of applying for a new job may take a moderate amount, as rejection from potential employers is a possibility and will require coping to respond positively. Taking a very ill pet that has been part of the family for years to the veterinarian to be euthanized would be taxing to the range and regulation of emotions.

Appropriateness of Emotions

The appropriateness of emotions is the affect and display of feelings during engagement in occupations (WHO, 2001). *Affect* is the physical display of emotions, usually portrayed in facial expressions. For example, when we are happy, we usually smile. This is a behavior that reflects our emotions. Regulating how we express our emotions is often required for activities that involve other people or when there are social expectations. For example, when playing a game, a child (or an adult for that matter) must learn to control her reactions when she loses or things do not go as planned (Figure 6-11). This is when it will be important for you to have already examined what the social demands are for the activity that you are analyzing. What are the common social expectations? Of course, we can all probably think of an example in which we saw someone demonstrate poor behavioral regulation (think about the fights you have seen or heard about at children's soccer and football games between parents). How many times have you wanted to laugh during a church service or at a time when it was definitely not appropriate to do so? You were utilizing behavioral regulation to downplay your display of emotions during those times.

The amount of appropriate display of emotions required of an activity is very much based on the social demands of the activity and the chance of error or negative incidents. Is there a chance that the person engaging in the activity will be faced with opposing views, a negative outcome, or errors? Will the person be faced with the possibility of not getting what he had expected or wanted (think of a child in a toy store)? Are there other people involved in this activity that expect certain emotional behavior? (For example, the actors involved in the Academy Awards are expected to act happy for their fellow nominees when they themselves do not win an award.)

Experience of Self and Time

Appropriateness and Range of Emotion

The function of experience of self and time also includes the range of emotions and the appropriate demonstration of those emotions. Refer to the previous section under "Emotional Function" for a description of *appropriateness of emotion* and *range of emotion*.

Body Image

Body image is related to a person's awareness of the physicality and image of his or her own body (WHO, 2001). This includes understanding what he or she looks like and his or her own height and weight. This comes into play in choosing clothing or activities to participate in. This is not an awareness of physical ability but having an understanding of one's own body parts and shape. This mental image of what one looks like is often disrupted when an amputation or a disfiguring accident occurs.

In determining if this factor is demanded of an activity, think about how the size or shape of the person is important to the activity. Is it important that the person have an accurate understanding of his or her size and shape? Is it important that the person have a concept of what he or she looks like? Does the person need to understand what attributes he or she has and what parts make up his or her entire body? Will an understanding of his or her body image shape his or her actions? Perhaps there are social demands of the activity that require an awareness of body image (such

as bikini modeling—anyone can wear a bikini, but our society demands a particular body shape for this).

Self-Concept

Having a self-concept is being aware of your roles and identity in the world. This goes beyond understanding how you look, which is addressed in body image; this is addressing who you are and what you understand about your position in the environment (WHO, 2001). Much of what you do every day as an OT student stems from an understanding of who you are as a person and what you believe your role in the world to be. You woke up this morning and made decisions based on this understanding of yourself (like reading this fantastic book). A mother wakes up every day with the understanding that many of the activities she must engage in address her role as a caregiver toward a child.

Therefore, in determining if self-concept is required of an activity, think about whether or not the activity is linked to a social or familial role. Does the activity require that the person understand and know what roles she plays in her environment? Does the activity require that she have a good understanding of who she is and how she relates to others (e.g., understanding gender, age, socioeconomic status)? For example, for a person to attend a support group for women who are divorced, she must first be able to identify herself as having those traits.

Global Mental Functions

Consciousness

Awareness and Alertness

The ICF defines *consciousness* as "the state of *awareness and alertness*, including the clarity and continuity of the wakeful state" (WHO, 2001, p. 48). The term *consciousness* is often used in medical facilities to describe a person's level of wakefulness. Consciousness is very much linked to arousal and, in definition, sounds similar. Consciousness is being awake, while arousal level is being able to respond to stimuli in the environment. There are varying levels of each, with people who waver in and out of consciousness (appear to be in and out of sleep), and there are varying levels of alertness, from slow to respond to a very heightened state (like someone who has just drank a cup of coffee and is directing a movie). We all function on

GLOBAL MENTAL FUNCTIONS	DESCRIPTORS
Consciousness	Awareness and alertness, clarity and continuity of the wakeful state
Orientation	Orientation to person and self, place, time, and others
Temperament and personality	Extroversion, introversion, agreeableness, and conscientiousness; emotional stability; openness to experience; self-expression; confidence; motivation; self-control and impulse control; appetite
Energy and drive	Motivation, impulse control, appetite
Sleep	Physiological process

a daily basis while conscious, so most activities will require this function. However, the level of arousal will vary depending on the demands of the activity (how quickly we need to respond to stimuli in the environment).

Clarity and Continuity of the Wakeful State

Being in an aroused or *wakeful state* is the ability to demonstrate alertness and respond to stimuli present in the environment (Buckley & Poole, 2004). The rapidity with which a person must respond to stimuli and the number of stimuli presented often determine the level of arousal required for an activity. For an activity in which constant diligence and quick reactions are expected, a high level of arousal is required. An example of this might be playing a game of tennis. The person engaged in the game must be on constant alert as to where the ball is going. There are many activities in which we engage every day that demand very little arousal. For example, many people get up in the morning, turn off their alarm clocks, take a shower, and get dressed while still half-asleep (low level of arousal or wakeful state).

In determining how much of a continuous wakeful state is required for an activity, think about how alert people must be to things that may occur in the environment. Does the activity require that they react quickly (such as with driving)? Does the activity span over a long period of time where a certain level of arousal must be sustained (sitting through a long lecture)? Does the activity occur at a time when alertness and arousal might be challenged, such as late at night or very early in the morning?

Orientation

Orientation to Person and Self

Being oriented to the *self or person* includes having an awareness of one's own identity (WHO, 2001). This means that the client understands what his or her name is and has an idea of who he or she is in relation to others. This differs from self-concept, which entails understanding who one is in society and having a concept of one is as a whole. In most tests for orientation, being oriented to the self entails being able to know your own name (Zoltan, 2007).

Orientation to Place

Orientation to place requires being aware of one's own location. This could include understanding the type of place one currently is in (home, hospital, or hotel), as well as in what city, town, or country (WHO, 2001). It is important to note that this differs from topographical orientation, which is the ability to follow a route or navigate through a physical environment to get from one place to another, such as riding a bike from home to a local grocery store (Zoltan, 2007). Orientation to place does not include this type of navigation ability but is simply the understanding of current location. This factor is required of activities that are context-specific, meaning that a specific environment is required of the activity in order for it to be successful. For example, one must be in a bathroom and understand that he or she is in a bathroom in order to be successful at the activity of toileting. Another example might be ordering food in a restaurant. It will be essential for the person to understand that he or she is in a restaurant in order to be successful at ordering food.

Orientation to Time

Being aware of the current date, month, day of the week, and year are all part of being oriented to time (WHO, 2001). This also includes having an awareness of approximately what time of day it is. This function is utilized during activities surrounding the environmental conditions, such as an understanding of what time of year it is to determine what clothing to wear. Having an awareness of what year it is also helps shape activities and interactions with others. While working in a nursing home years ago, I met a resident who was convinced that it was 1962 and that she needed to catch a bus to work. Every morning she would try to get out of the front door of the nursing home, screaming that she was going to miss her bus. She was obviously having difficulties with orientation in time (and also place). Our self-care activities are often shaped by an understanding of what day of the week it is, such as delaying or eliminating certain tasks on weekends, when they don't have to be done.

Orientation to Others

This mental function includes being aware of the identity of significant people in one's life (WHO, 2001). This includes being able to not only name a significant person in your life, but also to identify who he or she is in relation to you. For example, if your mother were to walk into the room, you should be able to identify that she is your mother. If a coworker walked up to you, you should be able to identify that he or she is a coworker, not your brother or sister. This is often a challenge for a person who experiences a brain injury or certain types of dementia, in which he or she mistakes a friend for a sister (or, even worse, his or her spouse). Of course, this function relies heavily on memory and perceptual functions (being able to remember names and relationships and also being able to perceive faces and voices).

Being able to identify others is important in activities that involve others or that are oriented toward others. For example, if a person is writing a letter to her old roommate from college, she must understand who that person is in relation to her. It would be an unsuccessful activity if she were to write the letter as if writing to her girl friend from high school. Of course, this factor is of utmost importance in interacting with others. It is demanded during activities in which certain social responses are expected of the person engaged in the activity. Perhaps how one behaves toward others is determined by having an understanding of each person's identity.

Temperament and Personality

Extroversion, Introversion, Agreeableness, and Conscientiousness

The mental functions of temperament and personality are defined as the "disposition of the individual to react in a particular way to situations, including the set of mental characteristics that makes the individual distinct from others" (WHO, 2001, p. 34). This includes specific personality traits such as extroversion, introversion, agreeableness, and conscientiousness. In analyzing an activity, certain personality traits are required at varying levels for certain activities. For example, a person who is extroverted is very outgoing and readily engages with others. People who work in sales, especially in retail or street markets, must be outgoing and demonstrate the trait of extroversion. The opposite of this is the introverted personality. Such people tend to be more focused on the self and internal thoughts and feelings versus those of others. These are people who tend to be labeled as "shy." Agreeableness is a trait that is characterized by being easily pleased and conforming to other's needs. This trait is especially helpful in activities where groups of people must come to a consensus or agree on an idea. A person who demonstrates conscientiousness is someone who is very careful and particular and governed by principles and a strong sense of what is right. Activities that require a strong sense of values and principles and put heavy ethical responsibilities on the participant will require a conscientious personality.

Emotional Stability

Emotional stability is characteristic of a personality and temperament that is "even-tempered, calm and composed" (WHO, 2001, p. 50). This type of temperament might also be termed *easygoing*. This function allows for interactions and actions that are not laden with irritability or anxiety. The type of temperament or personality a person has is an interesting concept to think about in analyzing the demands of an activity. Does a person need to be easygoing to complete the activity? For the answer to be yes, it most likely will be an activity that entails working with other people, with difficult issues, or in situations that require a calm environment. For example, in order to lead a relaxation group, the leader would need to

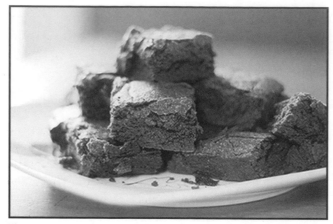

Figure 6-12. Impulse control: Brownies may be the ultimate challenge.

demonstrate the ability to relax and must have a calm demeanor (no high-energy or pressured behavior will help the group relax).

Openness to Experience

Being open to experience is a personality trait that allows a person to be accepting of new experiences and activities. This may also include controversial or surprise events that occur within a familiar activity. This requires that the person see new experiences as learning experiences or as opportunities to expand the self. Activities that fall outside of daily routines require openness to experience. Traveling to another country is an example of an activity where openness to experience is required.

Self-Expression

The ability to express one's feelings and emotions is an aspect of a person's temperament that allows for personal expression during activities. For example, many artists use self-expression in their work—a painter may use her inner feelings to design meaningful works of art. This is also a function required of personal conversations and expression to others in relationships. For example, during a disagreement with her significant other, Julie must rely on self-expression to get her true feelings across.

Confidence

Confidence is the belief in oneself, or being self-assured. People who have confidence will demonstrate that they will succeed in the venture ahead of them or the roles they inhabit. Activities that are especially challenging or have high social demands often require a high level of confidence. For example, interviewing

for a job promotion requires that the applicant demonstrate a high level of confidence. Every day, we see people engaging in activities that require confidence. A person who speaks to the manager of a department store about getting a return for a purchase must have some level of confidence in himself and what he feels is right.

Motivation

Motivation is the internal incentive to behave in a certain way or to take action (WHO, 2001). This is what often drives us to participate in activities that are beyond our basic needs. It is what allows us to do more than what is needed just to survive. As a personality function, being internally motivated is a temperament or personality trait. This is what drives some people beyond basic needs and to excel at those things that require a high level of motivation, such as obtaining a degree.

Self-Control and Impulse Control

Humans learn how to resist internal urges to do or say things from an early age. We learn that there are social demands of many of the things we do every day that do not allow for acting upon spontaneous needs or feelings. For example, we learn as children that although we may have an intense itch in a private area of the body, we are to resist the impulse to scratch while out in public. This is the impulse-control function at work. One must exercise impulse control when on a diet and someone offers freshly baked brownies. The amount of impulse control required of an activity is greatly influenced by the person engaged in the activity. If a person does not like chocolate, passing up a freshly baked brownie may not take much impulse control (Figure 6-12). However, there are many common traits that allow us to generate estimates of the amount of impulse control required of common activities. For example, maintaining a diet is an activity that, for most people, typically requires a great degree of impulse control. Controlling our impulses when we are around others is something that becomes automatic as we mature and come to understand social expectations. For example, during the activity of eating a meal with others, the impulse to belch out loud must be suppressed. Impulse control might also be exercised during this activity in selecting food and resisting the temptation to take more than a fair share of a certain food item so that the others at the table will also get enough to eat.

Appetite

Our natural desire for things is created by our appetite function. Natural desires are aspects that are physiologically driven (such as the desire for food or water) but are also driven by our psychological mechanisms (WHO, 2001). This is what drives us toward satisfying certain needs. This addresses a person's natural desire for certain sensory stimuli, such as the longing for touch. Appetite is often what drives us toward action. It is required of activities such as eating, drinking, smoking, drinking alcohol, sensory stimulating behaviors, and other physiological urges.

Energy and Drive

Motivation

As mentioned earlier, motivation is the internal incentive to behave in a certain way or to take action (WHO, 2001). This is what often drives us to participate in activities that are beyond our basic needs. It is what allows us to do more than what is needed just to survive. Our basic self-care needs require minimal motivation to complete. Higher motivation levels are required to complete tasks that have fewer rewards or are greater challenges. For example, if you are reading this book, you are motivated to achieve success in your OT program. You needed a certain level of motivation to even apply to OT school. Thus, in determining if motivation is required of an activity, think about what intrinsic or extrinsic rewards there are for engaging in the activity. Basic needs such as breathing and eating require very little motivation, as these activities are essential to life. However, greater internal motivation is needed to engage in activities that may not be immediately rewarded or may require a great amount of effort (like going to school to earn a degree). If a person is offered a million dollars to run around the block naked, he or she needs less internal motivation as he or she has an external motivator—the money. However, this person would need to be internally motivated by money in order for this to work. Either way, the person has to be motivated toward one thing or the other—toward the money or the idea of running around the block naked for the sake of doing it.

Impulse Control

See "Self-Control and Impulse Control," discussed on page 98.

Appetite

See "Appetite," discussed previously on this page.

Sleep

Physiological Process

Sleep is a mental function that entails "physical and mental disengagement" from the immediate environment (WHO, 2001, p. 52). Sleep as a physiological process is accompanied by changes in breathing and heart rate, as well as alterations in brain activity. This function is required only of the activities surrounding going to sleep. Thus, dreaming and sleeping are the primary activities in which this factor is required. It is important to note that this factor does not involve the amount of sleep a person achieves and how it affects participation in an activity. For example, it is tempting to state that sleep is required in order to drive long distances. However, the physiological process of sleeping during the activity of driving would be very dangerous (no sleeping at the wheel). Instead, the level of consciousness and arousal are factors that are in high demand for long-distance driving.

Complete Activity 6-1 to review this section.

SECTION 2: SENSORY FUNCTIONS

Visual Functions

Quality of Vision

The ability to detect light, contrast, and color among visual stimuli is one of the basic foundations of seeing functions. It is what gives us varying levels of visual acuity, being able to make out and detect various shapes of objects. Detecting light and contrast is what allow us to see words on a page (Figure 6-14), see a dog running across the street, or distinguish the face of a friend. Being able to detect color influences the choices we make between one item and another. Quality of vision is required in varying degrees for many daily activities. Activities that require minimal levels of visual acuity are many of the basic self-care tasks that utilize larger objects and employ many of our other senses. For example, when you shower and wash your hair, you are utilizing your sense of touch and proprioception to supplement your vision. You

ACTIVITY 6-1
REVIEW OF MENTAL FUNCTIONS

Identify how each of the following functions is utilized while buying a snack out of a vending machine (Figure 6-13). Assume that you are already standing in front of the machine with change in your pants pocket. Leave a row blank if a factor not used. In the final columns, indicate the extent to which each body function is challenged during this activity.

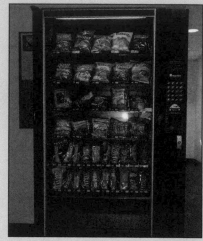

Figure 6-13. Vending machine.

SPECIFIC MENTAL FUNCTIONS	NONE	MINIMALLY CHALLENGED	GREATLY CHALLENGED	HOW IT IS USED
Higher-level cognitive				
Attention				
Memory				
Perception				
Thought				
Sequencing complex movement				
Emotional				
Experience of self and time				
GLOBAL MENTAL FUNCTIONS				
Consciousness				
Orientation				
Temperament and personality				
Energy and drive				
Sleep				

SENSORY FUNCTIONS	DESCRIPTORS
Visual	Quality of vision, visual acuity, visual stability, visual field
Hearing	Sound detection and discrimination, awareness of location and distance of sounds
Vestibular	Position, balance, secure movement against gravity
Taste	Qualities of bitterness, sweetness, sourness, and saltiness
Smell	Sensing odors and smells
Proprioceptive	Awareness of body position and space
Touch	Feeling of being touched, touching various textures
Pain	Localized and generalized pain
Temperature and pressure	Thermal awareness, sense of force applied to the skin

must see enough to get into the shower and where your supplies are.

Visual Acuity

Visual acuity is what allows us to detect form and contour—to see things clearly near and far. We use visual acuity to detect objects, differentiate between them, and discern details. We use acuity to read, find objects, and identify people in our environment. In determining if acuity of vision is needed for an activity, first think about what parts of the activity require that the person see something in the environment on which he or she must act, or what aspects of the activity the person must see while he or she is conducting the activity. For example, while driving, a person must be able to see and detect everything in the environment in order to react accordingly, using the controls of the car (e.g., steering, gas, or brake). There are activities that require detection of the person's actions in order to influence further actions, as in writing or typing. In writing by hand, the person must watch what he or she is writing and where he or she is headed on the page. While typing, the person may watch to see that what he or she hoped to type actually showed up on the page and respond by deleting unwanted characters or continuing on.

The amount of challenge that an activity brings to this function depends on the level of acuity required. What amount of detail must be detected? For example, reading the fine print on the packages of many medications or threading a needle would require a high level of visual acuity.

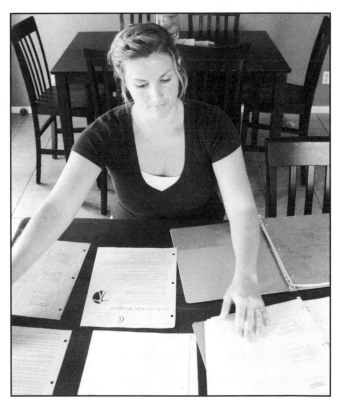

Figure 6-14. Reading requires a high level of quality of vision.

Visual Stability

Visual stability refers to our ability to perceive objects or our environment as stable (or not moving) even though our eyes are moving rapidly. These rapid movements of the eyes, called *saccades*, allow us to scan an environment or object (e.g., when reading) (Chang & Ro, 2007). Anytime we move our eyes

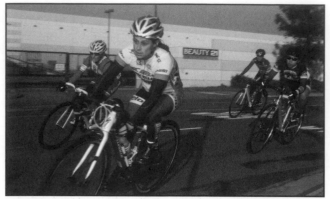

Figure 6-15. Riding a bike in the city requires visual stability.

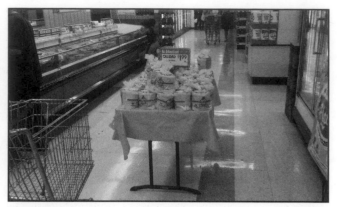

Figure 6-16. Awareness of objects in our visual field allows for safe navigation in environments like a grocery store.

rapidly and smoothly from one point to another, we are challenging our brain's ability to process what is moving and what is not. This allows us to determine if the environment is moving, if we are moving, if our eyes are moving, or if all three are moving. It becomes especially challenging when our bodies are moving and our eyes are also moving. This takes place in many sport and activity leisure activities, such as bicycling. When riding a bike, one must visually scan the environment for hazards and to make decisions as to where to steer. The cyclist is also moving within the environment. The sense of visual stability is what allows the cyclist to understand visually what is moving in the environment and what is not (Figure 6-15).

Visual Field

Visual awareness of the environment includes detection of all within the visual field: objects close to our body and those far away. The visual field includes all that we can see ahead of us, as well as on the periphery while still looking ahead (WHO, 2001). Without a full visual field, we would view the world as if looking through a tunnel. What we see in the periphery gives us additional information about the environment and may prompt us to action. For example, in walking through a grocery store while shopping, we walk through crowds and aisles in stores, using what we see in our periphery to avoid collisions. We also need to be visually aware not only of what is directly in front of us, but also of what lies ahead in the distance. This is visual function in action (Figure 6-16).

To determine if visual awareness at various distances is required of an activity, think about the environment in which the activity typically occurs. Where does the person engaging in the activity need to look? Does he or she need to be aware of the full environment? Does the person need to focus on objects near

and far? Does the activity require that the person be aware of all visual stimuli entering the environment? An example would be the activity of playing baseball. The players in the game need to be able to be aware of where the ball and other players are in the environment in all areas of the visual field. Without this, a player may be hit by a ball (or another player).

Hearing Functions

Sound Detection and Discrimination

During our daily activities, we hear and respond to certain sounds, based on our ability to detect noise. We discriminate between the pitch and volume of sounds to determine what is making the noise (Figure 6-17). Using this information, we respond. For example, we might respond to the sound of a child screaming in the street outside if the pitch and sound were of an urgent nature and not just playful. It is this ability to discriminate between sounds that allows us to act appropriately and safely within our environments. When determining if detection and discrimination of sounds is required of an activity, think not just of what noises occur during the activity, but also what noises require the participant to act upon the noises based on their ability to discriminate what is making the noise. For example, during the activity of washing hair, there are noises that occur, but none of them require the participant to discriminate and act upon the noises.

Awareness of Location and Distance of Sounds

Part of hearing functions is the ability to be aware of the location and distance of sounds. This is utilized

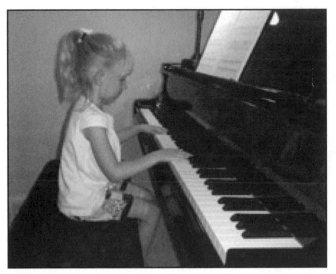

Figure 6-17. Playing the piano requires that the participant be able to detect and discriminate between different sounds.

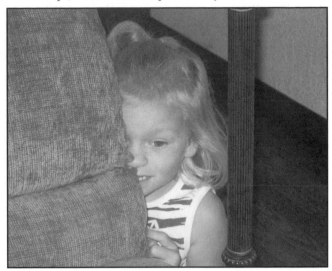

Figure 6-18. Using the ability to locate and determine the distance of sounds while hiding during a game of hide and seek.

when locating where a sound is coming from and approximately how far away it is. When driving, how do we know an ambulance is headed our way? Our first signal is the sound of the siren. From the sound, we can determine if the ambulance is behind, in front, or to the right or left of us. By the volume level, we can determine approximately how far away it is. The same is true of many sounds that we encounter in our daily lives. Think about how you know someone is approaching you from behind or coming down a hallway. As a child, if you ever played hide-and-seek, you utilized this hearing function as you listened for the footsteps and movements of your seeker as you hid (Figure 6-18). You might have even used this function as you took your turn as the seeker, trying to listen for the slightest sound made by those who were hiding. If you heard the floor creak or a tiny giggle, you would need to use your hearing functions to determine where the sound came from.

While many activities create noise or have sounds that occur during the activity, not all activities demand the use of this hearing function. To determine if this function is required, think about what sounds occur naturally in the environment in which the activity takes place. Are there noises that the person engaging in the activity must be able to identify and tell from which direction they are coming? Do sounds surrounding the person contribute to his or her understanding of what is going on around him or her? An example of this would be walking through a street fair where the noises from different directions tell the person what is occurring nearby. Also ask yourself if

the sounds he or she hears help determine action, as in the case of an ambulance, where the direction and distance of the siren sound will tell nearby drivers when they must pull out of the way.

Vestibular Functions

Position

Position is the sensory function of the inner ear that helps to determine the position of the body (WHO, 2001). For example, without the use of sight, it allows you to know whether you are sitting upright or leaning to one side. Because this function relies on the inner ear, the position of the head provides information on the position of the body. Thus, position is determined by the position of the head. In determining whether this is required, ask yourself the following: Does the position of the head change during the activity, and does the activity require the person to maintain a position? Does the person need to maintain the body in a particular position without using the sense of sight?

Balance

Balance is the body's ability to maintain an upright position while standing, sitting, or moving (*Stedman's Medical Dictionary*, 2012). The body's ability to maintain balance is also related to the functions of the inner ear. When one moves or is pushed or moved by an outside object, the ability to remain upright depends on the inner ear's ability to tell the brain and body how to stay upright. Just as with the position function, the

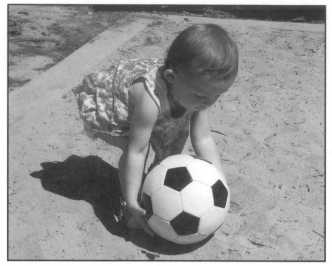

Figure 6-19. June picking up a ball from the ground, which challenges her balance.

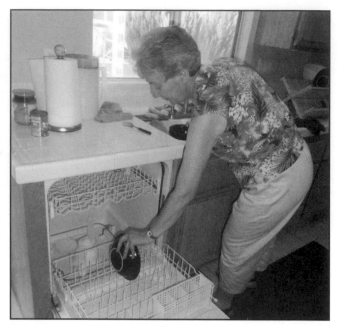

Figure 6-20. Sensation of securely moving against gravity: bending over to load the dishwasher.

position of the head provides the needed information about where the body is and how to maintain it in an upright position. Thus, any time the head is moved, this sense of balance keeps one from falling over. Balance will be required in any activity that requires bending over or changing head position or has the potential for an outside force pushing against the body. For example, June picking up a ball from the ground requires her to use her balance to keep from falling over (Figure 6-19).

Secure Movement Against Gravity

The vestibular sense is what allows people to move their bodies in the surrounding space against the forces of gravity. Without this vestibular sense, people would not be able to move about in their environment. It is this sense that enables people to be aware of their body position and maintain balance. The vestibular sense relies on the workings of semicircular canals of the inner ear, which sense the position of the head, changes in the speed at which the body is traveling, and changes in direction (Dunn, 2009). Having a sense of direction and upright position is foundational to postural control. It is what tells you which way is up or down as you position your body. When you stand up from a seated position, your vestibular sense tells you that you are moving upward and indicates when you have achieved an upright stance. Without this, you might lean to one side or fall over. You might also feel as if you were moving when you are not. So in any activity that requires the body to move forward, backward, up, down, or side to side, this factor will be

required. It is especially challenged during activities in which balance is needed or when vision is occluded. We use our vision to supplement our vestibular sense in telling us direction and position in space. For example, if you were to bend over to tie your shoes, you would watch your surroundings change as you bent forward, telling you that your position had changed. This, combined with your vestibular and proprioceptive sense, would allow you to bend forward without falling over and to come back up to a standing position when finished. If you were to do this with your eyes closed, you would be relying only on your vestibular sense to tell you where you were in relation to gravity and your proprioceptive sense to tell you where your limbs and trunk were in relation to each other (Figure 6-20).

In determining if vestibular factors are required of an activity, think about how much the body and head move during the activity. Does the activity require that the person stand and move about? Does the activity require the person to lean forward outside of his or her center of gravity? Does the activity challenge the person's balance, perhaps with limited visual input? Is the body moving forward or side to side, in which case the person must determine speed of movement? Does the person's position in space determine further action? An example of this would be if the person were climbing a ladder; in that case, the position of the body would determine each subsequent movement. Does the position of the head change during the activity, such as leaning the head back while showering to rinse shampoo out of the hair?

Taste Functions

Qualities of Bitterness, Sweetness, Sourness, and Saltiness

The ability to taste is a function in which chemicals reaching the taste buds are broken down into signals representing bitterness, sourness, saltiness, and sweetness (Dunn, 2009; WHO, 2001). While the discrimination of each of these tastes relies on the perceptual abilities of the brain (discussed earlier in this chapter), taste functions depend on the ability of the tongue to detect chemicals and send neural signals regarding each of the chemicals on to the brain. Taste functions come into play with activities surrounding eating or drinking or any activity in which there will be contact with the tongue. This function is highly challenged in those who must determine differences in ingredients or the level of sweetness or bitterness in foods, as in the case of a chef or wine critic. For most of us, some level of taste function is required to motivate us to eat or drink and to determine if an item we are ingesting is safe to eat. This relies on the brain's ability to perceive the signals it receives regarding these different foods.

Smell Functions

Sensing Odors and Smells

Sense of smell is the ability to sense odors and smells in the environment (WHO, 2001). The sense of smell requires the nose to perceive chemicals in the air and send signals regarding these chemicals to the brain. It is here that smell is perceived and the type of smell is distinguished (see perceptual functions discussed earlier in this chapter). Smells can be associated with objects, environments, people, or situations. The sense of smell has been linked to memory and emotion (Dunn, 2009). Smells can alert us of situations that require action, such as a bad body odor or the smell of smoke. Odors can also be soothing and comforting or can cause discomfort. The sense of smell is required for activities that give us information regarding the environment. We need to be able to detect changes in the environment and to tell whether such changes call

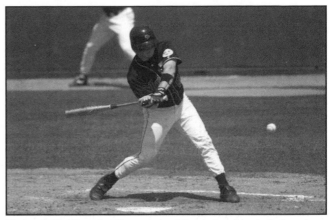

Figure 6-21. When holding a bat while playing baseball, the player must use his ability to determine where his body is in space.

for action (e.g., the dog relieved himself in the corner of the kitchen).

Proprioceptive Functions

Awareness of Body Position and Space

The ability to determine where one's body parts are moving and in which direction they are moving or being held is controlled by sensory receptors in our muscles, tendons, and joints (Dunn, 2009). Muscle spindles are the sensory components that detect muscle length, telling us how much a muscle is stretched or contracted. Golgi tendon organs receive information about joint movement by detecting the movement of tendons that surround the body's joints. These two sensory receptors send information, creating an awareness of where each body part is in relation to the others and within space (WHO, 2001). To understand what these signals mean, this sense also requires the perceptual abilities of the brain to interpret the information sent from the proprioceptive receptors in the body.

All activities that require movement utilize the proprioceptive sense to some degree. Activities that occur outside of the range of sight require a higher level of this factor, as the person must rely on his or her ability to sense where a body part is instead of seeing it. An example of this is in playing baseball or softball (Figure 6-21). When a person is standing holding a bat, the bat is held up and behind the head. It is the proprioceptive functions that provide information regarding the position of the body and how the bat is positioned.

Touch Functions

Feeling of Being Touched

Touch is the ability to perceive contact with the skin or mucous membranes (*Stedman's Medical Dictionary*, 2012). The ability to determine when we are being touched is employed throughout many of our daily activities and often occurs without our awareness. As you sit reading this book, you are aware of how the book is touching your skin and how it is lying in your hands. Any time you come in contact with an object or something is placed against you or into your mouth, you are drawing on your ability to be comfortable with and understand the sensation. We act on and respond to touch, depending on the type of touch and where we are being touched. For example, this sense is helpful in knowing when there is a spider or bug crawling on your skin. It is the touch functions that notify you that your clothing needs to be adjusted (such as an unbuttoned sleeve or the shoulder strap of a dress) or if you need to wash your hands after working in the yard.

If the activity you are analyzing requires contact with others (such as a hug, holding hands, or even bumping into each other in passing) or contact with objects, this factor is utilized. Also, think about what type of clothing or equipment must be worn on the body. Touch also comes into play when one is eating food and being able to recognize when and where there is still food in the mouth. Being able to recognize items by touch of the fingers or hand is essential to much of what we do. For example, when you type on a keyboard, you are using your sense of touch to determine where the keys are. Because we utilize our hands for so much of what we do, in conducting an activity analysis, think also about what the hands come in contact with during the activity. Does the person need to determine when and where an item is being touched or an item is touching them?

Touching Various Textures

Touch functions include not only the ability to recognize when and where one is touched, but also to differentiate various textures. This includes being able to distinguish one texture from another and tolerate the texture. We use this ability every day without recognizing it. When you hold this book and turn the pages, you are using your ability to feel the pages as you turn them. When you button your shirt or pants, you use your sense of touch to discriminate between the edges of the buttons and the buttonholes. Your touch functions also allow you to discriminate between rough and smooth, allowing you to be comfortable with objects and different textures touching your skin. Any time you come into contact with an object or something is placed against you or in your mouth, you are drawing on your ability to be comfortable with the sensation and to regulate it. Without this, you would have difficulty wearing clothes, washing yourself, and even brushing your hair. Objects and materials that come into contact with our bodies come in a variety of consistencies and textures. For example, the texture of sandpaper is one that, for most people, is not a sensation that is comfortable against the skin. Many people feel the same about softer, slippery substances, such as the skin of a slug or frog.

In determining the extent to which touch functions are used, think about how much the person comes into contact with different textures. Does he or she need to act according to what is being felt (as when buttoning a button, using the sense of touch to feel the edges of the button)? Does the person need to be able to tolerate different textures? For example, to scuba dive in cold water, one must be comfortable with a wet suit covering and pressing against one's body. There is also a face mask pressing against the skin and sand against the feet and between the toes.

Pain

Localized Pain

Being able to identify when potential or actual damage may be occurring in a part of the body and where it is occurring is essential to maintaining your own safety. Localizing where the pain is coming from requires the functioning of pain receptors in the body part that is receiving the insult. These signals allow us to quickly know which part of the body is in danger and react by pulling away or caring for the injury. It is pain that alerts us that something is wrong and tells us to act. For example, as Richard is out gardening and picking raspberries, he feels a sharp pain in one of his fingers (Figure 6-22). Upon inspection, he finds that a small splinter has lodged itself under the skin in his finger. The area continues to hurt, so he promptly pulls the splinter out and washes the area. Without the signal that the splinter was there, the area would have become infected, and he could have eventually lost the finger to amputation—all from a simple splinter. It is discomfort that causes you to change position and even to shift in your seat after sitting for a long time.

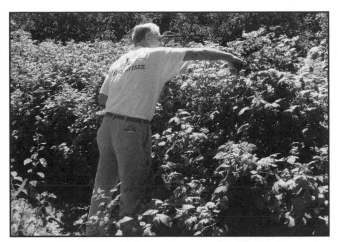

Figure 6-22. Being able to detect injuries using our sense of pain is useful when engaging in activities such as picking raspberries.

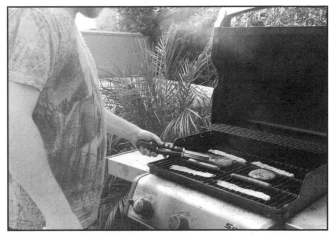

Figure 6-23. Thermal awareness, or awareness that heat is being used when cooking at a barbeque grill.

Without this feeling of discomfort, you might sit for hours in one position, putting you at risk for sores on the backside. Notice how many times you shift in your seat as you continue to read on.

Activities that utilize this function are ones in which action is required in response to discomfort and being able to determine where on the body the pain is coming from. The pain might be a limiter, telling the person to stop a particular action or keeping the person safe during the activity. An example of this would be lifting a heavy object. Does the activity present the chance of injury? Does the environment in which the activity commonly occurs have elements that could cause harm? For example, hiking in the woods occurs in areas where branches and plants can cause scratches and animals can bite.

Generalized Pain

Generalized pain is pain that occurs in nonspecific areas and is focused in larger areas. An example of this is the pain experienced throughout the body when one has the flu. Generalized pain provides us with information regarding the body and any dysfunction that may be occurring. Generalized pain indicates the need to rest or to provide additional care to the body. These signals are helpful during activities where the body may be pushed to extremes. For example, if you are hiking at a high elevation, you might begin to experience bodily discomfort due to the lack of oxygen to your systems and brain. Generalized pain is not commonly involved in most activities but is essential to the maintenance of daily health.

Temperature and Pressure

Thermal Awareness

Another sensation that alerts us to possible harm is thermal awareness, which is the ability to sense heat and cold (WHO, 2001) (Figure 6-23). You may use a part of your body to feel if an object is hot or cold, such as feeling the temperature of bath water before stepping into it or placing gloves over your hands when you sense that it is very cold outside. These sensations guide our actions and choices in tasks (to place gloves on or not). We use this sensory function when eating as well (determining if what we are eating is hot or cold).

To determine if this function is demanded of an activity, think about what objects and materials are involved in the activity. Does the person interact with or touch those objects? What is the typical environment of the activity? For example, if walking across the beach, it will be important to know how hot the sand is before walking across it barefoot. Thus, think about the effect the environment might have on a person's body or on objects.

Sense of Force Applied to the Skin

The ability to feel pressure against the body differs from the sense of touch. The receptors within the body that detect pressure differ from those of touch and serve a different purpose. Force or pressure against the skin can be felt in varying degrees, with corresponding implications. How strongly an

Activity 6-2

Review of Sensory Functions

Identify how each of the following functions is utilized while buying a snack out of a vending machine. Assume that you are already standing in front of the machine with change in your pants pocket. Leave a row blank if a factor is not used. In the final columns, indicate the extent to which each body function is challenged during this activity.

SENSORY FUNCTIONS	NONE	MINIMALLY CHALLENGED	GREATLY CHALLENGED	HOW IT IS USED
Visual				
Hearing				
Vestibular				
Taste				
Smell				
Proprioceptive				
Touch				
Pain				
Sensitivity to temperature and pressure				

item is being grasped, how tight the fit of pair of pants is, or if a watch band is strapped on too tightly can be detected using the sense of force or pressure. To determine if the sense of force on the skin is required during an activity, ask yourself at what times pressure is being applied to the person or whether the person is applying pressure to an object. Does he or she need to regulate that pressure?

Complete Activity 6-2 to review this section.

Section 3: Neuromusculoskeletal and Movement-Related Functions

Joint Mobility

Joint Range of Motion

The ease with which a joint moves through motion is termed *range of motion* (WHO, 2001). The degree to which range of motion is required of an activity calls for careful analysis of all of the movements that

NEUROMUSCULOSKELETAL AND MOVEMENT-RELATED FUNCTIONS	DESCRIPTORS
Joint mobility	Joint range of motion
Joint stability	Maintenance of structural integrity of joints

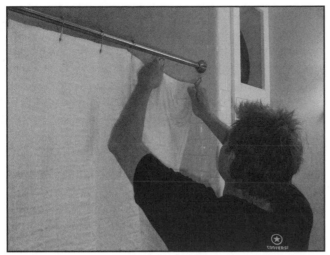

Figure 6-24. Reaching up to hang a shower curtain requires a great amount of joint range of motion in the shoulders.

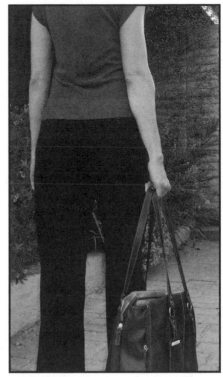

Figure 6-25. Carrying a heavy bag can be a strain to joint stability.

typically occur during the activity. It is important to consider the demands on all of the joints in the body: fingers, spine, hips, knees, and ankles, just to name a few. An understanding of what comprises a full range of motion for each joint will enable you to determine the extent to which each joint is challenged. For example, regarding normal range of motion, consider the fact that maximal flexion is approximately 180 degrees. In analyzing the activity of placing cups in a cupboard that is at eye level, we find that this activity challenges shoulder flexion only moderately. Hanging a shower curtain would pose a maximal challenge for shoulder flexion for a person of average height (Figure 6-24). Be sure to consider both ends of the range (both flexion and extension), as some activities require greater extension than flexion; for example, playing tennis requires full elbow extension.

One should also be careful not to confuse range of motion with strength. Neither the weight of the objects used nor the number of repetitions is of importance here. Range of motion is not a consideration of muscle strength but of the ability of the joint to move smoothly. To determine the extent to which this factor is utilized, identify which body parts move and which are attached to the joints, allowing them to move. To what extent is each joint moved through its potential range of motion? Is the body part moved minimally and thus through smaller degrees of movement or does the body part move toward the end ranges of flexion or extension?

Joint Stability

Maintenance of Structural Integrity of Joints

The stability of a joint is what allows for its proper alignment. Stability is a function of the joints' structural integrity (WHO, 2001). It is the structure and stability of the joints that keep bones in proper alignment, allowing for functional use of the body parts and trunk. Without this, our limbs might land outside of alignment or put extra strain on other parts. Examples of when joint postural alignment goes awry include shoulder dislocations and spinal scoliosis.

The alignment of joints is challenged in activities that stress the stability of a joint. Having proper joint alignment will be important in activities if a joint is to be moved through more than a minimal range of motion. It is also needed if stress will be placed on the joint, as when a heavy bag is being carried in the hand, causing stress on the joints of the fingers as well as the shoulder (Figure 6-25).

MUSCLE FUNCTIONS	DESCRIPTORS
Muscle power	Strength
Muscle tone	Degree of muscle tension
Muscle endurance	Sustaining muscle contraction

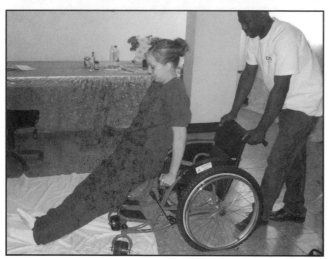

Figure 6-26. Pushing the body up in a wheelchair requires a great amount of muscle power.

Section 4: Muscle Functions

Muscle Power

Strength

The force with which a body part must move or hold an object requires the functions of muscle power. An activity may require the power of one muscle, a group of muscles, or muscles throughout the body or trunk. This includes maintaining postures (e.g., the muscle contractions required to maintain an upright stance). Muscle power requirements vary according to the environmental challenges and exertion against gravity. For example, walking up a steep hill requires a greater amount of strength than does walking on a flat surface. The amount of muscle strength required will be much less if gravity is being used as an assist, such as reaching down to the ground, versus moving against the forces of gravity, such as standing up from the floor. The muscle challenge may come from moving the weight of an object or moving the weight of the body, as in doing a push-up (Figure 6-26).

There are times when detailed analysis of exactly which muscles are used during an activity is required. This has been termed *muscular analysis* and is also utilized by other disciplines, such as physical therapy (Bukowski, 2000). Being able to dissect the movements required into the exact muscles utilized during an activity requires a knowledge of kinesiology. It is beyond the scope of this book to go into detail regarding anatomy and kinesiology. It is important, however, to be able to identify the major muscle movements. It is through muscular analysis that clinicians often find "just-right challenge" for a client. If you were working with a client who needed to strengthen his or her wrist supinators, how would you decide on an activity that would help with this? Clinicians must often mentally analyze the muscular demands of several activities to find one that will meet the need. Muscular analysis is also helpful in gaining awareness of the activities with which your client might have difficulties, given a certain deficit of muscle power. For example, if you had a client with weakness in elbow flexion, you might think about the basic self-care skills involving elbow flexion that your client might find difficult (self-feeding, brushing teeth, pulling up pants).

It is important to recognize each of the movements required and the demand on the muscles not only for the upper extremities, but also for the trunk, hips, and lower extremities. Refer back to the steps that you found were needed to complete the activity. In steps where the body is used to support or move an object or the body must hold itself up against gravity, you would need to determine what types of muscle contractions had occurred—isometric, isotonic, or eccentric. Isometric contractions occur when there is no actual movement but muscles are contracting in order to hold a body part or joint in place (Breines, 2009). You utilize isometric contractions when you are holding this book. To hold the book still, you must use the muscles in your hands and perhaps other muscles in your upper extremities, depending on whether you have the book set on a surface or not.

ACTIVITY 6-3

MUSCULAR ANALYSIS

Identify how each of the following functions is utilized while buying a snack out of a vending machine. Assume that you are already standing in front of the machine with change in your pants pocket. Leave a row blank if a factor is not used. In the final columns, indicate the extent to which each of the body functions is challenged during this activity.

MUSCLES	NONE	MINIMALLY CHALLENGED	GREATLY CHALLENGED	HOW IT IS USED
Shoulder flexion				
Shoulder extension				
Shoulder abduction				
Shoulder adduction				
Shoulder internal rotation				
Shoulder external rotation				
Elbow flexion				
Elbow extension				
Wrist supination				
Wrist pronation				
Wrist flexion				
Wrist extension				
Thumb flexion				
Thumb abduction				
Finger flexion				
Finger extension				
Trunk flexion				
Trunk extension				
Trunk rotation				
Lower extremities				

You utilize isometric contractions of these muscles to hold the book in a static position. If you were to lift the book up, you would be creating an isotonic contraction. This is when muscles actually shorten during the contraction (Breines, 2009). Even without lifting an object, any movement that requires the muscle to shorten would be considered an isotonic contraction. Eccentric contraction occurs when this tension is released and the muscle becomes elongated. For example, if you were to set this book down on the ground, your biceps would contract and then slowly release as you gradually lowered the book to the floor. Because gravity is helping to pull the book toward the floor, the biceps would still be contracting to hold it up but would slowly be releasing their contraction to allow your arm to straighten. You would not be using the triceps to extend the arm unless you were forcefully throwing the book to the floor (which I do not recommend). Determining which type of contraction occurs will help to indicate the extent to which muscle power is needed for the activity you are analyzing (Activity 6-3).

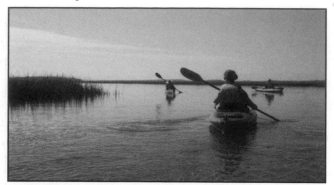

Figure 6-27. Kayaking for long distances requires muscle endurance.

Muscle Tone

Degree of Muscle Tension

Muscle tone is the natural tension that is present in muscles when at rest. This tension is what creates resistance or the lack of resistance when a body part is moved passively (WHO, 2001). Normal tone is required to allow for smooth muscle control (Preston, 2009). In order for muscles to work together to move a body part, one must work as the agonist muscle and contract while the opposite muscle, the antagonist, must allow for passive movement. For example, in bringing a spoon to your mouth, your biceps shorten while the triceps elongate. If the triceps had abnormally high tone, the biceps would find it more difficult to flex the elbow smoothly.

Normal tone is necessary for activities in which a muscle will be passively stretched. For example, if you were reaching down to your feet in order to tie your shoes, the muscles in your back would have to have a normal level of tone to provide some resistance, but not so much as to prevent you from flexing your trunk forward. Normal tone is also a prerequisite for smooth movements. Think about when you take a drink from a cup. You pick it up and slowly bring it to your mouth. If your tone is normal, the triceps elongates nicely and your biceps continues on its course in curling the cup toward your mouth. However, if your triceps was hypertonic or had fluctuating tone, it might cause the muscle to contract, thus extending the arm, and then the biceps would try to continue in its course by flexing the arm, so you now have the drink all over your lap. So think about how essential smooth movements are to the activity you are analyzing.

Muscle Endurance

Sustaining Muscle Contraction

Muscle endurance is required when the contraction of a muscle must be maintained for a prolonged period of time (WHO, 2001). Activities such as standing for long periods or holding an extremity in a static, isometric contraction, such as in carrying a box, both require muscle endurance. The longer the muscle is required to maintain a contraction, the more endurance is in demand. Muscle endurance could also be required when repetitive muscle contractions occur over a long period of time with minimal or no rest breaks (Figure 6-27). For example, painting a house requires the endurance of upper extremity muscles to repeat the same motions over and over again.

To determine the extent to which muscles are challenged to sustain contraction, take a look at the steps required of the activity—how long do some of the steps last? Do some of these steps require continuous action of the same muscle groups? Does the person stand or use trunk muscles throughout? Are there rest breaks during the activity? This would reduce the demand for muscle endurance. If many muscles are used during the activity and there are no certain muscles or muscle groups that must sustain a contraction, this function is not required or is minimally challenged.

SECTION 5: MOVEMENT FUNCTIONS

Motor Reflexes

Involuntary Reflexes: Involuntary Contractions of Muscles Automatically Induced by Stretching

Reflexes are motor movements and responses to sensory stimuli. A stretch reflex occurs when a muscle is stretched to the point at which an involuntary contraction of the muscle is induced (WHO, 2001). This is a protective response of the muscle to prevent overstretching. It is controlled by receptors in the muscles, called *muscle spindles*, which send signals to the spinal cord regarding the length of the muscle (Preston, 2009). This occurs without the person's

MOVEMENT FUNCTIONS	DESCRIPTORS
Motor reflexes	Involuntary reflexes: involuntary contractions of muscles automatically induced by stretching
Involuntary movement reactions	Postural, body adjustment, and supporting reactions
Control of voluntary movement	Eye-hand and eye-foot coordination, bilateral integration, crossing midline, fine and gross motor control, oculomotor control
Gait patterns	Movements used to walk

intent or involvement. The stretch reflex is utilized during activities in which muscles are stretched to end ranges. Our stretch reflexes prohibit stretching the muscles too far. Yoga is an example of when this protective reflex is utilized, during movements requiring deep stretches. This function will be utilized only if there is a chance of muscles being stretched to great lengths. For many sporting activities, this reflex often prevents injuries.

The asymmetrical tonic neck reflex (ATNR) is a primitive reflex that is present in infants and disappears by 3 to 4 months of age. This reflex serves a good purpose in those first few months of life in that it prevents an infant from rolling over before it is motorically and neurologically ready (*Mosby's Dictionary of Medicine*, 2006). When the head is turned to one side, the extensor tone on the side toward which the person is facing increases and the flexor tone on the opposite side increases (Preston, 2009). So, if an infant turns its head to the right, the right arm will extend and the left will flex (Figure 6-28). The occurrence of this reflex in an adult is not normal and can interfere with functional movements. Thus, ATNR will not be needed for the activities of an adult and will only be utilized only as a protective reaction in infants up to 4 months of age.

The symmetrical tonic neck reflex (STNR) is also a primitive reflex that is helpful only in infants and recedes after the first year of life. The STNR causes two different actions with head flexion and extension. With head flexion, the upper extremities go into flexion and the lower extremities into extension. When the head is extended, the upper extremities go into extension and the lower extremities into flexion (Preston, 2009). This is often called the *crawling reflex*, which allows infants to get into the crawling position (*Mosby's Dictionary of Medicine*, 2006). This reflex

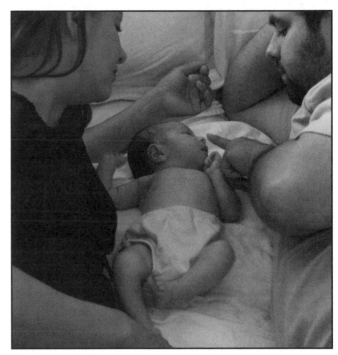

Figure 6-28. A baby exhibiting the ATNR reflex.

does not allow for actual crawling but lets an infant get into the quadruped position. This factor will be functional for infants only during the first year of life.

Involuntary Movement Reactions

Postural Reactions, Body Adjustment Reactions, and Supporting Reactions

Our bodies have natural reactions that are designed to protect us and allow us to restore our bodies to a natural upright position. When we sense that our balance is threatened or that we might be falling, our bodies automatically react to restore alignment of the trunk by increasing tone in the trunk or limbs (WHO,

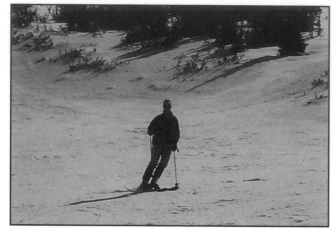

Figure 6-29. Skiing demands many involuntary movement reactions.

2001). These automatic reactions to being thrown off balance are often what keep up from falling. We do this by moving our feet or legs, extending our arms to help to regain balance, and shifting the head in a direction that will assist in regaining balance.

This function is especially important during activities where there is a chance of the position of the body being suddenly shifted. If a person's body is thrown or shifted from an upright position by another person, object, or the environment, he or she will utilize righting reactions to keep from falling and to regain an upright position. An example of how the environment can often challenge this factor is during snow skiing (Figure 6-29). As skis go over different terrains, the body is shifted in different directions and often thrown outside of its center of gravity. The skier's body automatically contracts muscles to help maintain an upright position. Without this, with every little bump that the skier goes over, he or she would find him- or herself tumbling down the hill. Righting reactions are also utilized any time the body is moved from the upright position, as in getting up from the ground (much as the skier would have to do if he or she tumbled down the hill) or in coming up from a supine position, such as lying in bed.

This function is required if sudden unexpected events cause a person to be thrown off balance or shifted from an upright position. Think about the environment in which the activity occurs—are there obstacles or other people that could cause a shift in balance? Does the activity require that the person reach outside of the center of gravity or bend downward and then regain an upright position? Think about the various positions that the person will be in during the activity and if the person must regain an upright position.

Control of Voluntary Movement

Eye-Hand and Eye-Foot Coordination

Moving in simple and complex ways requires coordinating many different body functions. Eye-hand or eye-foot coordination requires utilizing what is visually perceived in the environment to contract and control muscle groups to move in a coordinated fashion (*Stedman's Medical Dictionary*, 2012). For example, when you reach for your toothbrush, you are using visual information to control how and where to reach. In placing toothpaste on the toothbrush, you are again coordinating what you do with your hands with what you see to make sure that the toothpaste ends up on the toothbrush and not in the sink.

We utilize this connection between visual stimuli and movement in all activities where there is visual information that guides our movements. Handwriting is an example of using eye-hand coordination. We use this connection in many everyday self-care activities, such as grabbing toilet paper, scooping up food in a spoon, and washing our hands. The level of challenge to this factor comes with the demand for precision of movements and timing. For example, catching a quickly moving ball requires a high level of eye-hand coordination owing to the timing of coordinating movements with the visual stimuli of the moving ball.

Eye-foot coordination functions in the same way, coordinating what is visually seen with what the lower extremities are doing, as when kicking a ball or pushing the brake in a car in response to a small child running across the street. The demand for precise movements is another reason there might be a high level of eye-hand coordination needed. For example, threading a needle requires very precise hand movements using the visual stimuli of the direction of the thread as it is aimed toward the small hole of the needle. In determining whether this factor is utilized or not, think about how much the person must visually attend to an object or environment in order to guide his or her movements. If the steps can be done out of sight or without visual information, eye-hand coordination is not essential to the task (Figure 6-30).

Bilateral Integration

Bilateral integration occurs when both sides of the body, arms, or legs, are used collaboratively to complete a task (*Stedman's Medical Dictionary*, 2012). One extremity can work in conjunction with the other actively or as an assist. When both extremities are

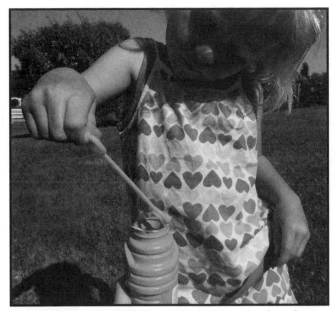

Figure 6-30. Playing with bubbles requires precise eye-hand coordination.

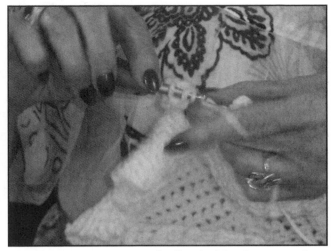

Figure 6-31. Knitting is an example of how both hands must coordinate movements together.

actively involved in the activity, each hand, arm, or leg has its own actions that work in collaboration with the other. An example of this is opening a jar or bottle: one hand grasps the bottle while the other twists off the lid. If it is collaborating passively, a limb may be used to stabilize an object while the other one is active. An example of this is writing. The nondominant hand holds the piece of paper down while the other hand does the writing. In the case where the bilateral coordination consists of one extremity being a stabilizer, the level of challenge is low, as there is little to no movement required of one extremity. Higher-level challenges occur when both hands and their fingers have individual movements. An example of this is in tying one's shoelaces or knitting (Figure 6-31).

To begin to understand whether this factor is used in an activity, begin by thinking about what objects are manipulated or moved by either the arms or the legs. Does it take the use of both sides? Do the hands have to work together to complete the steps of the activity? Perhaps the lower extremities must work together to manipulate an object. Does an object need to be stabilized while the other extremity does more of the action involving the object? Is each hand performing separate movements (indicating higher demand)?

Crossing Midline

The midline is the imaginary line that runs through the center of the body, dividing it into right and left halves (*Mosby's Dictionary of Medicine*, 2006). Crossing midline occurs when the right side of the body crosses over into the left side's territory or vice versa. When a person uses his or her right hand to brush the left side of his or her head, he or she crosses midline. If we reach with our right hand to pick up a cup that is on our left side, we are crossing midline. Any time our extremities or trunk cross over into the opposite side, the muscles of our trunk must collaborate with the movement of our extremities. Using the example of reaching to the left to grab a cup, our trunk muscles must contract and turn the trunk to the left to allow the hand to reach the cup. Crossing midline may not require the trunk to twist or even move, but it may require the trunk to contract muscles in order to stabilize and keep the body from tipping over. This all occurs without our awareness but allows us to dynamically interact with the surrounding environment. Without this, we would conduct only those tasks that were within reach, in a static position, not reaching across the body or leaning to either side.

Activities that require crossing midline require dynamic movement of the trunk and movements of the extremities toward the opposite side. Imagine a line down the center of the body. During the activity, does the right side ever come over into the left side, or the left into the right? This includes areas of the trunk that shift from midline. Does the activity require reaching? Does the activity require the legs to cross over one another? Think about the direction of the head—does it cross over into one side or the other?

Fine Motor Control

Fine motor movements are those that utilize the smaller muscles of the hand, fingers, and thumb.

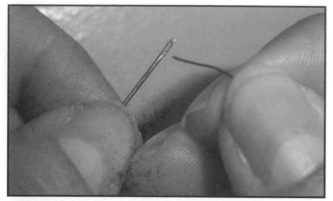

Figure 6-32. Threading a needle requires a great amount of fine motor control.

These muscles allow for the precise movements used to manipulate smaller objects. This includes picking up and releasing small objects, grasping objects with the hand (such as a doorknob), and pinching something between the thumb and fingers. The extent to which fine motor control is utilized during an activity is greatly influenced by the size and shape of objects used in the activity. For example, in the activity of dressing, there is greater challenge if a person is dressing formally in a dress shirt with small buttons and pants with a zipper versus the little fine motor needed to don a T-shirt and sweatpants. Fine motor control will still be utilized to put on these simpler clothing items when pinching and grasping the material to pull it on the body.

Most fine motor movements require the use of the hands. Fine motor movements will be required of any activity that uses the hand to grasp and release an object. The grasp may require all of the fingers to work together with the thumb, as in picking up a ball, or use individual fingers, as in holding a key. The extent to which fine motor movements are challenged is determined by the size and shape of the objects used and the demand for precision in the movements. To again use the example of threading a needle, very precise movements are required to move the thread into a very small hole (Figure 6-32). Fine motor movements occur not only when there is an object to grasp, but also when individual finger movements are required, as in playing a musical instrument like the piano or guitar. Individual finger and thumb movements are also required in typing on a keyboard and using a cell phone. Without these precise movements, we might be sending strange text messages to the wrong people.

Gross Motor Control

Gross motor control exists when the larger muscles of the body are used to coordinate movements. Actions such as throwing, jumping, or kicking are examples of gross motor movements. Gross motor movements are also considered larger movements, without the demand for small and precise control of actions. These larger movements typically use the larger muscles of the body, such as the quadriceps, biceps, triceps, deltoids, and pectoral muscles (this is just a few of the many possible). Gross motor movements can also utilize smaller muscles when done in combination with each other. An example of this is when the finger flexors of the hand are contracted to create a "gross grasp," wherein there is no specific prehension pattern because there is no isolated contraction of one of the smaller muscles of the hand. Movements of the trunk are also considered gross motor movements, as they utilize larger muscles and typically produce larger, less precise movements. The speed at which the limb or trunk is moved is also part of gross motor control. We utilize gross motor control throughout our daily activities. It is what allows us to bring food to our mouths without spilling it. We use it to guide our limbs into clothing and to move our arms in styling our hair. Without gross motor control, we might actually find that we were hitting ourselves or making a mess while doing these activities. If you were to try brushing or combing your hair with jerky arm movements, you would probably end up with a very wild hairstyle.

To determine if gross motor control is utilized during an activity, think about the movements made during the activity. Are they broad and large or small and precise? Think about what joints are moving—are the joints controlled by larger muscles like the shoulder, hips, knees, or elbows? How much does the trunk move? How much do the gross motor movements need to be coordinated and have few extraneous movements? There are some activities that are very forgiving in the amount of coordination needed, whereas other activities require a greater level of accuracy in movements. For example, washing a car utilizes large movements of the arms to move the sponge across the surface of the car, without any need for exact coordination of movements. However, when a person is picking up a glass and placing it in a cupboard (Figure 6-33), greater accuracy of movement is required or the glass will hit the cupboard or another glass and shatter. Think about how quickly the limb or trunk must move and then slow down—does this regulation of speed influence success? For example, if swinging a bat to hit a baseball, one must coordinate a quick contraction of the arms and trunk but then conclude the contraction very quickly. This is also part of gross motor control—being able to start and stop contractions at the appropriate time as well as to control the speed at which the limb is moving. To what extent would extraneous movements interfere with success in this activity?

Oculomotor Control

Motor control of the eye muscles allows for the detection of visual information in the environment and requires multiple types of coordination. *Saccades* are rapid eye movements from one aspect in the environment to another, without movement of the head or body (Zoltan, 2007). Moving our eyes from one point to another smoothly allows us to gather information about the world around us. For example, as you read this sentence, your eyes are moving smoothly across the page and seeing each word. When your eyes reach the end of a line, they swiftly and smoothly shift to the left and down to the next line. Reading is a perfect example of when saccadic eye movements are required.

Another type of oculomotor control is *pursuits*. This is where the eyes follow a moving object and keep it in focus (Zoltan, 2007). For example, to look at a bird flying in the sky, the muscles in your eyes must work to move along with the bird to keep it in your sight. Thus, the term *pursuits* is fitting, as the eyes are pursuing or chasing a moving object. Examples of activities that utilize this are watching or playing a sport, playing with a dog, or playing a video game.

Accommodation occurs when the eye muscles must coordinate to allow for looking at objects near and far or when an object is changing distance from near to far (or vice versa) (Zoltan, 2007). Our eyes accommodate to the changing distance; they must focus when we take notes in class in front of us and then look up at the instructor in front of the class. Our eyes must refocus at a different distance. This also occurs when we are visually attending to an object that is traveling toward or away from us. An example of when this occurs continuously is when a person is driving. We see cars approach us while others move away.

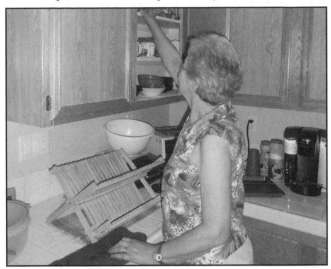

Figure 6-33. Using large muscles to control where dishes go in the cupboard.

Oculomotor control has the challenging task of binocularity, where it must coordinate the movement of two eyes in exactly the same way in order to maintain view of an object. That means that if you were watching a car that was traveling left to right, both your eyes would have to be fixated, following the car at the same rate. Without coordination of both of the eyes, we see double (which is called *diplopia*) (Warren, 2009). Paralysis or changes in the muscle tone of one eye can cause difficulty in the ability to move both eyes in the same manner. The ability to coordinate the eyes together is what allows us to accurately determine where an object is in space. It provides us with information as to the distance and placement of objects. For example, when we reach for a cup sitting on a table, both of our eyes focus on it and we reach forward based on the visual information we receive on where it is—to the left or right and how far forward. A person with double vision or the lack of binocularity might see two cups and have a misperception of how far away the cup was. He or she might grasp too close or too far away and knock the cup over.

To determine if oculomotor control is utilized during an activity, think about how much visual tracking and focus is required. Does the activity require that the person look at objects, either stationary or moving? Does it require that the person look across the environment, moving the eyes in a swift but coordinated manner (e.g., when reading)? Is the perception of depth or position important? Think about the objects that are used or are part of the environment—are the

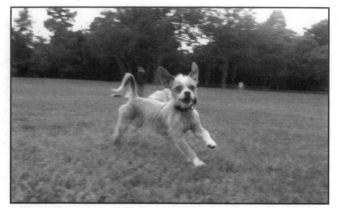

Figure 6-34. Following a running dog involves oculomotor control.

eyes required to move in order to see these objects (Figure 6-34)? Does the person need to look near to far or see objects as they move closer? To what extent do smooth movements of the eyes influence success in this activity? How much is coordination of the eyes challenged during the activity to move smoothly at the appropriate rate?

Gait Patterns

Movements Used to Walk

Gait patterns are related to the movements used to walk. These patterns are important to OT practitioners in how they relate to the ability to engage in occupations. Thus walking in a grocery store or during the preparation of a meal is within our domain, while the simple action of walking without engagement in an occupation is not. A normal gait pattern includes the use of both legs interchangeably, shifting body weight from one leg to the other (Bolding, Adler, Tipton-Bruton, & Lillie, 2009). This requires coordination of each leg to swing forward as the other leg maintains

balance. The cadence or rate in which all of this occurs is also a component of normal gait patterns.

In analyzing the demand for gait patterns in an activity, the first step is to determine if any walking is required, and if so, how much. How important is it that the person have a "normal" gait pattern? The purpose of the walking, as well as the social demands surrounding the activity, may be what determines the extent to which a normal gait pattern is required. For example, a person who decides to do runway modeling will definitely need to walk with a certain gait pattern. Distance and terrain of the environment may also challenge the need for gait patterns. If a person is hiking up a mountain, a higher-level gait pattern would be required than would be needed to walk in a grocery store.

Complete Activity 6-4 to review this section.

SECTION 6: CARDIOVASCULAR, HEMATOLOGICAL, IMMUNOLOGICAL, AND RESPIRATORY SYSTEMS FUNCTIONS

Cardiovascular System Functions

Blood Pressure

Blood pressure is the amount of pressure that is exerted by the blood on the walls of the veins and arteries of the body. This pressure is regulated by the amount in which the heart muscles contract, the volume of blood in certain areas of the body, and the contraction or dilation of the arteries (*Mosby's Dictionary of Medicine*, 2006). For example, when one has been sitting for a long time, blood tends to

CARDIOVASCULAR, HEMATOLOGICAL, IMMUNOLOGICAL, AND RESPIRATORY SYSTEMS FUNCTIONS	DESCRIPTORS
Cardiovascular system	Blood pressure, heart rate and rhythm
Hematological and immunological systems	Hematological and immunological systems
Respiratory system	Rate, rhythm, and depth of respiration
Additional functions of the cardiovascular and respiratory systems	Physical endurance, stamina, aerobic capacity

ACTIVITY 6-4

REVIEW OF NEUROMUSCULOSKELETAL AND MOVEMENT-RELATED FUNCTIONS

Identify how each of the following functions is utilized while buying a snack out of a vending machine. Assume that you are already standing in front of the machine with change in your pants pocket. Leave a row blank if a factor is not used. In the final columns, indicate the extent to which each body function is challenged during this activity.

FUNCTION	NONE	MINIMALLY CHALLENGED	GREATLY CHALLENGED	HOW IT IS USED
Joint mobility				
Joint stability				
Muscle power				
Muscle tone				
Muscle endurance				
Motor reflexes				
Involuntary movement reactions				
Control of voluntary movement				
Gait patterns				

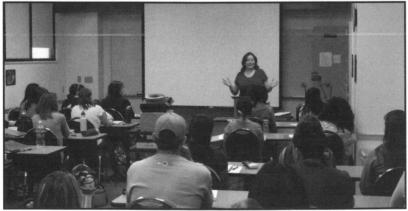

Figure 6-35. Giving a speech may challenge heart rate and blood pressure.

pool in the legs. When you stand suddenly, your body must work hard to maintain proper blood pressure or you might feel dizzy from a reduced supply of oxygen to the brain (this is called *orthostatic hypotension*—decreased blood pressure when changing position). Blood pressure normally increases with activity as the heart pumps harder and faster. Blood pressure can be challenged by physical and psychological stresses. For example, heart rate and blood pressure may be challenged when you are digging in the garden a

of a large audience
al response to stress-
you are giving a speech the autonomic nervous
(Figure 6-35). The heart rate, blood pressure, and
ful situations is White, 2009).
system, which of blood pressure is essential to
other body how much it is challenged during an
d on many factors. Activities in which
A of the body changes rapidly will challenge
's ability to maintain normal blood pressure.

If you have ever been on a roller coaster that drops suddenly, you may have felt slightly light-headed as your body tried to regain normal blood pressure and oxygenation of the brain. Activities that may stimulate the autonomic nervous system will challenge blood pressure, as the body reacts to stressful situations. This can be positive stress, such as running a marathon or interviewing for a job. It can also be negative stress, such as being stuck in traffic on the way to the job interview.

Heart Rate and Rhythm

The function of the heart is to deliver blood to all areas of the body. The rate at which this occurs (how often the heart contracts) is based on the need for blood and oxygen to all areas of the body. Thus the heart will need to pump faster when there is a higher demand, as when the extremities are moving and require blood and oxygen to function. There are many factors that can contribute to a change in heart rate, including the autonomic nervous system and adrenaline. Typically, during activity, the heart rate should not exceed 20 beats per minute above the resting heart rate. Maintaining the heart rate needed to deliver the appropriate amount of blood and oxygen to the body is a function that is often challenged during activities that require a great amount of movement or varied amounts of movement, where the heart rate may need to fluctuate between high and low. Activities that challenge heart rate may also be those that stimulate the sympathetic nervous system through stressful situations. For example, in taking an exam or meeting someone you are attracted to, your heart rate may increase.

Having a heart that beats on a consistent basis is a necessity of living; however, the extent to which maintaining an actor obtaining a specific heart rate is required of occurs. relies on the context in which the activity will determine amount of physical challenge to the body will need to in amount by which the heart rate of the body. Does meet the circulatory demands stopping of movement require the starting and regulate the rate in fast and then return thus the heart needing to a psychological stressor pumping from slow to may challenge the heart to heart rate? Is there it is beating? the activity that te at which

Hematological and Immunological Systems Functions

Hematological System

The hematological system relates to the blood and the blood-forming tissues of the body, which include the bone marrow and spleen (*Mosby's Dictionary*, 2006). The primary function of blood is to carry oxygen and nutrients to cells within the body. Blood also carries away carbon dioxide and other waste to be removed from the body. Our blood transports hormones that signal other areas of the body into action. Blood also allows wounds to stop bleeding and send an immunological defense to fight infections. The hematological system is essential for survival and is challenged during activities that require efficient delivery of certain elements to parts of the body. An example of this would be delivery of electrolytes to muscles used during a physically strenuous activity. It is also required if there is risk of bruising or injury. If contact with objects occurs, the clotting functions of the blood allow physical contact with objects or other people that may cause bruising or abrasions without continuous bleeding.

Immunological System

The immunological system works to protect the body against infection and other pathological organisms and actions. The immunological system is composed of the bone marrow, thymus, spleen, and lymph tissues (*Mosby's Dictionary*, 2006). Immunology, the study of body's response to threats, is a complex and expansive area of human science. For the sake of activity analysis, the OT practitioner needs to have a basic understanding of how the immunological system plays a role in the engagement in activities. There are practitioners who specialize in this area and develop a deeper understanding of how the function or dysfunction of the immunological system can influence participation in occupations. An example of this is a practitioner who specializes in lymphedema management. In this area of practice, the clinician works with clients who are limited by an excessive accumulation of lymph fluid in a limb.

The immunological system is utilized in everyday activities, to a greater extent when confronted with environments that present hazards. For example, if sitting inside our one's home reading a book, one's immunological system is not challenged. However, if playing on the playground with other children, one's immunological systems must go to work to fight off the multiple viruses and bacteria one may be exposed to. When analyzing an activity and determining if the immunological system is challenged, think about the environment in which the activity commonly occurs. Does the activity occur outside of the person's home? Is there interaction with others? Does the person need to touch objects that have been touched by others or have been outdoors? How clean is the typical environment?

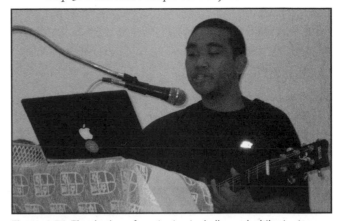

Figure 6-36. The rhythm of respiration is challenged while singing.

Respiratory System Functions

Rate of Respiration

Respiration is the process of moving air in and out of the lungs. The rate in which this occurs typically ranges from 12 to 20 breaths per minute in adults (*Mosby's Dictionary of Medicine*, 2006). The rate in which air is brought into the lungs is dependent upon the body's need for oxygen. Because oxygen is required for movement of the body, with increased movement there is an increased demand for oxygen. Thus, for activities that require great amounts of movement, the respiration rate increases to meet the demands. Slower rates of respiration may be required for activities focused on relaxation or sleep. The amount of oxygen available in the air may influence the rate of respiration as experienced in higher elevations. When the air in the environment contains a lower concentration of oxygen, the lungs must work harder to supply a sufficient amount of oxygen to the body. Thus activities conducted at higher elevations will require a greater challenge to respiratory rate.

Rhythm of Respiration

Respiratory rhythm is the cycle of inspiration and expiration of air from the lungs (*Mosby's Dictionary of Medicine*, 2006). A normal breathing pattern will match the demands for oxygen in the body. Abnormal rhythms are seen when there is a brief cessation of breathing when there is a need for oxygen in the body, during rapid cycles when at rest, or during ataxic breathing, where there are quick breaths alternating with slow ones. The demand for a specific rhythm of respiration increases as the demands for oxygen change. As a person starts to move or stops moving, the rhythm in which he or she is breathing should change accordingly. In activities where there is continuous movement, a respiratory rate that will allow the body to continue moving efficiently must be established. An example of this comes from long-distance running. Experienced runners learn to pattern their respirations so that they are breathing efficiently. The rhythm of respiration is challenged in other activities such as swimming, where there is a regular cessation of breathing followed by large inhalations. Rhythm of respiration is also challenged during singing (Figure 6-36) or delivering a speech. Activities that involve the production of speech or sounds via the mouth will include controlling respiratory rhythm. Eating also requires regulating the rhythm of respiration around swallowing of foods and liquids.

Depth of Respiration

Depth of respiration refers to the volume of air inhaled and exhaled (WHO, 2001). Shallow breathing occurs when small amounts of air are inhaled. Smaller amounts of inhaled air produce smaller amounts of oxygen distributed to the body. The depth of respiration is linked to the need for oxygen in other areas of the body. With greater demands for oxygen, respiration depth is greater. For example, when you are climbing a tree, your lungs will expand and inhale more deeply than when you are sitting and reading a book. The depth of inspiration can also be influenced by what will be done with the exhalation of air. Singing or playing a musical instrument such as a flute will require a deep inspiration, as the long and sustained exhalation will be utilized to create music.

To determine the extent to which this function is utilized, think about how much the body is moving. Does the body move over a period of time in which

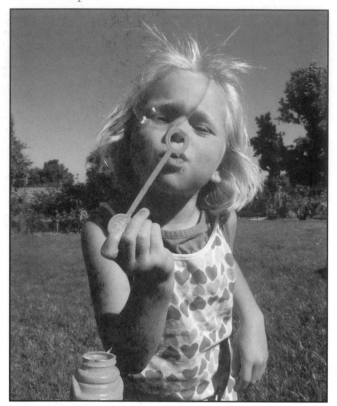

Figure 6-37. Blowing bubbles challenges depth of respiration.

blood will need to deliver adequate oxygen? This means that a simple short movement such as reaching for a book may not require deep respirations, but repeating this motion repeatedly would. Does the activity require use of air coming out of the body, such as blowing up a balloon, blowing bubbles (Figure 6-37), whistling, singing, or playing a wind instrument?

Additional Functions of the Cardiovascular and Respiratory Systems

Physical Endurance, Stamina, Aerobic Capacity

Endurance as it relates to the cardiovascular and respiratory systems involves continuous efficient action of the heart and lungs to provide oxygen to the body. Cardiac endurance requires that the heart maintain a rate and rhythm over time as the body moves throughout the activity. This is essential for activities that occur over a longer period of time with few breaks. This means that the heart and lungs must endure a certain pace and provide the necessary oxygen to the rest of the body as needed. It is this cardiac and respiratory endurance that often challenges many people

during aerobic exercise. Not only is muscle endurance required, but endurance of the heart and lungs is also needed to provide oxygen to those muscles.

Activities that utilize physical endurance and stamina require prolonged movement and increased respiratory and heart rates. Activities that require continuous movement with little to no rest breaks will challenge this factor. In analyzing an activity to determine if physical endurance is utilized, think about how much the person must stand or move. Are there any opportunities for break so the heart rate and respiratory rate will have a chance to lower to close to a resting rate? Are the heart and lungs required to maintain a particular rate for a prolonged period of time, such as in singing or swimming?

The ICF defines aerobic capacity as "the extent to which a person can exercise without getting out of breath" (WHO, 2001, p. 80). Reaching the point of being out of breath is determined by the efficiency in which the body is utilizing oxygen. When the body is not able to absorb and utilize the amount of oxygen needed, the body's natural reaction is to increase the respiration rate to increase the amount of oxygen the lungs are bringing into the body. Thus aerobic capacity is about the amount of physiological work the body must do in order to absorb oxygen. An activity that requires a high level of aerobic capacity is one that requires the body to efficiently absorb oxygen while moving for long periods of time. Aerobic capacity is required of all activities that call for long periods of movement and require sufficient delivery of oxygen to the limbs or muscles used. Hiking and long-distance bicycling are examples of situations in which aerobic capacity is challenged.

SECTION 7: VOICE AND SPEECH; DIGESTIVE, METABOLIC, AND ENDOCRINE SYSTEMS; AND GENITOURINARY AND REPRODUCTIVE SYSTEMS FUNCTIONS

Voice and Speech Functions

Voice functions are those that produce noise by sending air through the larynx (WHO, 2001). Humans use the noise that is produced as a primary mode of communication: speech. Without voice, our mouths

VOICE AND SPEECH; DIGESTIVE, METABOLIC, AND ENDOCRINE SYSTEMS; AND GENITOURINARY AND REPRODUCTIVE SYSTEMS FUNCTIONS	DESCRIPTORS
Voice and speech	Rhythm and fluency, alternative vocalization functions
Digestive, metabolic, and endocrine systems	Digestive, metabolic, and endocrine systems
Genitourinary and reproductive systems	Urinary functions, genital and reproductive functions

would move but nothing would be heard. Producing a voice requires a coordination of the respiratory system and the larynx and surrounding muscles. This coordination is what allows for volume, pitch, and resonance of a voice (WHO, 2001). Identifying the need for this function in activity is fairly easy in that if any talking is involved, it is needed. The extent to which this factor is challenged depends on the extent to which the voice is utilized—at what volume, at various pitches, and with what quality. Delivering a speech is an activity that requires a high level of voice functions, whereas an activity that requires a low level would be talking face to face with a friend or whispering to the person next to you in class.

Rhythm and Fluency

In order to be understood by others when we speak, a certain flow and tempo are used to express the beginning and ending of statements, emotion, and emphasis on specific words. For example, when one is telling a joke, the punch line is usually told with a certain intonation that indicates to the listener that those last few words are the highlight of the joke. The rhythm of our speech patterns also communicates to the listener the emotion behind what is being said. Rapid speech sends a message of urgency, while slow, deliberate speech communicates a more relaxed feeling (Figure 6-38).

Fluency is what allows us to speak one word after another fluidly and smoothly. Without this, we would stumble over words or repeat parts of words, as in stuttering. Being able to smoothly transition from one word to another is what allows us to communicate efficiently and effectively. This is especially important when we are trying to portray an urgent message or to communicate with those we do not know. For example, if you were calling a 911 operator, it would be imperative to be

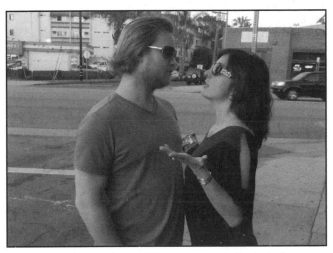

Figure 6-38. Voice and speech functions are challenged when communicating to others.

able to string together the words needed fluently and smoothly to communicate the facts of the emergency that is occurring. Rhythm and fluency are utilized in producing speech but are challenged when one is confronted with activities posing greater demands. When the expectations or needs of the listener are higher, the demand for rhythm and fluency increases.

Alternative Vocalization Functions

There are times when vocalizations are produced for activities outside of those involving speaking. Alternative vocalizations are those needed for yelling, singing, humming, chanting, or crying. Before a child gains the ability to speak, crying is its way of communicating. Even after learning how to speak, we continue to use alternative vocalizations for calling attention to others—by yelling. Singing, humming, and chanting are sustained vocalizations that produce noise but do not necessarily entail the use of words.

Activities that require alternative vocalizations are those in which typical speech is not utilized but the vocal cords are still used. Children and infants utilize this function in much of what they do during waking hours. Adults may communicate with infants in similar ways with coos and babbles. Laughter is considered an alternative vocalization that is utilized in many activities throughout the life span. These alternative vocalizations are still a means by which to communicate; they are simply ways of doing so without the use of words. Activities that utilize this function are those that demand or produce some use of the voice during the course of the activity. Children and infants will require this function as a way of communicate needs; when they are hungry or have a dirty diaper, they will cry. Communicating to others a sense of joy or happiness during an activity will require this function to produce a laugh or giggle. In situations where the attention of another or perhaps an animal is required, a loud noise or yell will be needed.

Digestive, Metabolic, and Endocrine Systems Functions

Digestive System

The digestive system is what allows for the transportation of food or liquids through the body, to be absorbed and broken down (WHO, 2001). When food is swallowed, it moves through the gastrointestinal system by movements called *peristalsis*. Peristalsis moves the food from the stomach and into the intestines. While food moves through each area of the gastrointestinal system, nutrients are absorbed from it and pass into the bloodstream. Activities that include eating or drinking will require use of the digestive system. Greater challenges to the system will be meals of greater size and complexity. For example, food items that are more difficult to digest (i.e., are denser in consistency) will pose a greater challenge to the digestive system.

Metabolic System

The metabolic system is what allows our bodies to utilize food and convert it to energy. This includes the breakdown and utilization of carbohydrates, proteins, and fats (WHO, 2001). This broad and basic definition does not fairly reveal the complexity of this system. However, the *Framework* states that as OT practitioners, we are to have a broad understanding of how this function influences engagement in occupation. As

mentioned earlier, there are clinicians who may choose to specialize in some of these functions, necessitating extra training and education. On a basic level, the metabolic system is utilized when the body needs to utilize food as energy. The greater the amount of energy needed, the greater the demand on the metabolic system to perform. For example, swimming requires energy supplied to the arms and legs in order to allow the muscles to contract. Without a source of energy, the muscles would be unable to move the limbs.

Endocrine System

Much like the metabolic system, the endocrine system is complex; it will get little time in the spotlight here and will require further inquiry for those involved in this specialty area. The endocrine system regulates hormone levels within the body, including growth and metabolic hormones (*Mosby's Dictionary of Medicine*, 2006; WHO, 2001). The glands and other structures that secrete hormones help regulate daily, monthly, and annual rhythms. These hormones are often what drive us toward certain actions and allow us to function from day to day. They give us drive toward reproduction, control the appetite, and allow mothers to produce milk while nursing their babies. Some hormones regulate the salt and water balance in the body when it is engaged in strenuous activity. These are just a few of the ways in which the endocrine system is utilized in activities beyond keeping the human body alive and healthy. Refer to the literature on endocrinology for a greater understanding of the scope of this system.

Genitourinary and Reproductive Systems Functions

Urinary Functions

Urinary functions are utilized for one purpose only—to release urine from the body (WHO, 2001). This includes controlling the release of the urine, which is called *continence*. The ability to refrain from releasing urine at inappropriate times is required for most activities, especially those around other people. This function is especially challenged when the person is required to go long periods of time before being able to urinate. An example of this might be if riding in a bicycle race. There would be minimal opportunity to relieve the bladder along the long trail. Urinary functions are especially in demand when urination is part of the activity, as when using the bathroom or if giving a urine sample while

ACTIVITY 6-5

REVIEW OF CARDIOVASCULAR, HEMATOLOGICAL, IMMUNOLOGICAL, AND RESPIRATORY SYSTEMS FUNCTIONS

Identify how each of the following functions is utilized while buying a snack out of a vending machine. Assume that you are already standing in front of the machine with change in your pants pocket. Leave a row blank if a factor is not used. In the final columns, indicate the extent to which each body function is challenged during this activity.

FUNCTIONS	NONE	MINIMALLY CHALLENGED	GREATLY CHALLENGED	HOW IT IS USED
Cardiovascular system: blood pressure, heart rate, and rhythm				
Hematological and immunological systems				
Respiratory system: rate, rhythm, depth of respiration				
Additional functions: physical endurance, stamina, aerobic capacity				

visiting the doctor. To determine the extent to which urinary functions are required of an activity, think about the context(s) in which the activity occurs and if there is opportunity to empty the bladder. How much time passes between the opportunities for this? Is the person required to hold his or her urine for long periods of time? Is urination part of the activity? Are there social demands of the activity that require the person be continent? Certainly a person in front of an audience must not relieve him- or herself while giving a speech.

Genital and Reproductive Functions

According to the ICF, the genital and reproductive functions include sexual functions, menstruation, procreation, and sensations associated with genital and reproductive functions (WHO, 2001). Sexual functions are related to the mental and physical aspects of performing sexual acts (WHO, 2001). These acts do not necessarily require the involvement of another person. The menstrual cycle is also controlled by the reproductive system and regulates the periodicity and extent of menstrual bleeding. Of course, this occurrence is experienced only by women. The ability to procreate or create and give birth to a child is also part of the genital and reproductive functions. Male and female fertility is required in order to create a fetus, followed by the woman's ability to carry the child in her uterus until birth. It is the genital and reproductive functions that give women the ability to produce milk for the child once born.

Activities that require genital and reproductive functions are those that include sexual activity incorporating the genitals. The genitals can be used for creating a child or for enjoyment only. If the purpose of sexual activity is to procreate, the demands on this function are greater, as fertility functions will be required. Any activity surrounding the menstrual cycle will also require this function, as with some self-care activities.

Complete Activity 6-5 to review this section.

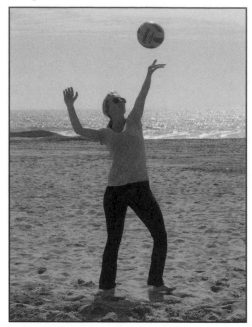

Figure 6-39. The protective functions of the skin allow us to interact with objects such as when hitting a ball during volleyball.

SECTION 8: SKIN AND RELATED STRUCTURES FUNCTIONS

Skin Functions

Protection

The skin is designed to protect us from physical, chemical, and biological elements that might cause harm to our bodies (WHO, 2001). This is especially important when we are surrounded by or come in contact with elements that, if they gain access to our bloodstream, would cause us harm. Our hands come in contact with bacteria and germs on a continuous basis, but the skin surrounding our fingers prevents these from entering our bodies. Protection fails when these elements are introduced to our mouths, nose, or cuts in the skin. The skin also shields us from elements of the environment such as wind, heat, cold, and sun. Environments that experience extreme temperatures or climates challenge the protective functions of the skin.

Any time we come in contact with an object or other person, the protective functions of our skin are utilized to protect us. The greater the amount of pressure or shearing forces, the greater the challenge is to this function. For example, if you were shoveling dirt in a

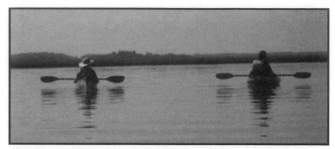

Figure 6-40. Repetitive motions such as rowing challenge the skin functions of the hands.

garden, the skin on your hands would be challenged to endure the shearing forces of the shovel handle against the skin. The environment is also a consideration in analyzing the extent to which this function is utilized. Is there extreme heat, where the skin is required to sweat? Is the skin exposed to sun or wind? Extreme conditions will challenge the skin to protect the inner temperature of the body (Figure 6-39).

Repair

Skin has the amazing capacity to heal itself. When damage occurs through tearing, ripping, cutting, or burning, the skin begins a process of repairing the wound. This process is required of activities in which maintaining skin integrity is important. As mentioned in the previous section, the skin serves to protect the body; otherwise it would be at risk for exposure to harmful elements. If an activity involves the chance of injury to the skin, the repair functions of the skin will be necessary. Activities that require a person to regain skin integrity in order to continue on with an activity will also utilize this function. An example of this would be the activity of participating on a rowing team. If a blister develops on a rower's hand, his or her wound-healing functions must quickly go to work to allow the person to get back to rowing on the team (Figure 6-40).

Hair and Nails

Growing hair and nails is a function of the skin and related structures. Growing either of these would not necessarily be required of an activity, but having hair or nails could be. The presence of hair or nails is required for certain tasks, such as brushing hair or trimming nails. Fingernails also provide support at the tips of the fingers when grasping objects. The absence or presence of either nails or hair can also

SKIN AND RELATED STRUCTURES FUNCTIONS	DESCRIPTORS
Skin	Protection, repair
Hair and nails	Hair and nails

ACTIVITY 6-6

REVIEW OF VOICE AND SPEECH; DIGESTIVE, METABOLIC, AND ENDOCRINE SYSTEMS; GENITOURINARY AND REPRODUCTIVE SYSTEMS; AND SKIN AND RELATED STRUCTURES FUNCTIONS

Identify how each of the following functions is utilized while buying a snack out of a vending machine. Assume that you are already standing in front of the machine with change in your pants pocket. Leave a row blank if a factor is not used. In the final columns, indicate the extent to which each body function is challenged during this activity.

FUNCTIONS	NONE	MINIMALLY CHALLENGED	GREATLY CHALLENGED	HOW IT IS USED
Voice and speech				
Digestive, metabolic, and endocrine systems				
Genitourinary and reproductive systems				
Skin and related structures				

---

be considered under the *body structures* section, discussed in the next chapter.

CONCLUSION

The *Framework* delineates that part of determining the demands of an activity include examining the body functions required. Body functions are the physiological aspects of the human body such as sensory, mental, neuromuscular, skeletal, and cardiovascular functions. Body functions are the features that reside within the client that influence skill level but do not assure a certain skill level. Skill level is influenced by many factors, such as the environment and the challenges of the activity. Engagement in an activity requires a complex interaction of many body functions. Activity analysis includes understanding the role of each of the body functions and the extent to which each is challenged during an activity. With this knowledge, the clinician can better understand what contributes or limits participation in occupations and can be used to develop strategies for intervention.

Complete Activity 6-6 to review this section.

QUESTIONS

1. What is the difference between judgment and cognitive flexibility?

2. In what activities is insight an important body function?

3. What is multisensory processing and why is it important?

4. Of the perceptual functions, which do you utilize the most when driving? When studying? When grocery shopping?

5. Which of the thought functions do you utilize the most when driving, studying, or grocery shopping?

6. What is the difference between emotional stability and coping?

7. Why would tolerance of ambient sounds be needed during activities?

8. Describe the function of awareness of body and space and how it is utilized. How is it different from moving securely against gravity?

9. What is muscle tone?

10. Name five activities that require bilateral integration.

11. In what types of activities would alternative vocalization functions be utilized?

ACTIVITIES

1. Continue to analyze the activity of washing hair in the shower by completing Activity 6-7.

2. Continue to work on the Occupation-Based Activity Analysis form from Appendix B on the occupation you have chosen. Complete sections 8 and 9.

3. Choose a specific mental function and global mental function and find an activity that challenges both. Complete an analysis of the body functions required of the activity using section 9 of the form in Appendix B. What additional sensory functions are required of the activity?

4. Complete an activity analysis of an activity in which you participate in every day. Using the activity analysis form in Appendix B, complete section 9 and identify which body functions are the primary functions utilized.

ACTIVITY 6-7

Determine the body functions required of washing hair in the shower as it typically is done. Describe briefly how each of the body functions is used and then indicate the extent to which each body function is challenged. If a body function is not used at all during the activity, check off "none" and leave that row blank.

FUNCTION	NONE	MINIMALLY CHALLENGED	GREATLY CHALLENGED	HOW IT IS USED
Specific Mental Functions				
Higher-level cognitive: judgment, concept formation, metacognition, executive functions, praxis, cognitive flexibility, insight				
Attention: sustained attention and concentration; selective, divided, and shifting attention				
Memory: short-term, working, and long-term memory				
Perception: discrimination of sensations–auditory, tactile, visual, olfactory, gustatory, vestibular, and proprioceptive				
Thought: control and content of thought, awareness of reality, logical and coherent thought				
Sequencing complex movement: regulating speed, response, quality, and time of motor productions				
Emotional: regulation and range of emotion, appropriateness of emotions				
Experience of self and time: appropriateness and range of emotion, body image, self-concept				
Global Mental Functions				
Consciousness: awareness and alertness, clarity and continuity of the wakeful state				

(continued)

ACTIVITY 6-7 (CONTINUED)

FUNCTION	NONE	MINIMALLY CHALLENGED	GREATLY CHALLENGED	HOW IT IS USED
Global Mental Functions				
Orientation: orientation to person and self, place, time, and others				
Temperament and personality: extroversion, introversion, agreeableness, and conscientiousness; emotional stability; openness to experience; self-expression; confidence; motivation; self-control and impulse control; appetite				
Energy and drive: motivation, impulse control, appetite				
Sleep: physiological process				
Sensory Functions				
Visual: quality of vision, visual acuity, visual stability, visual field				
Hearing: sound detection and discrimination, awareness of location and distance of sounds				
Vestibular: position, balance, secure movement against gravity				
Taste: qualities of bitterness, sweetness, sourness, and saltiness				
Smell: sensing odors and smells				
Proprioceptive: awareness of body position and space				

(continued)

ACTIVITY 6-7 (CONTINUED)

FUNCTION	NONE	MINIMALLY CHALLENGED	GREATLY CHALLENGED	HOW IT IS USED
Sensory Functions				
Touch: feeling of being touched, touching various textures				
Pain: localized and generalized pain				
Temperature and pressure: thermal awareness, sense of force applied to the skin				
Neuromusculoskeletal and Movement-Related Functions				
Joint mobility: joint range of motion				
Joint stability: maintenance of structural integrity of joints				
Muscle Functions				
Muscle power: strength				
Muscle tone: degree of muscle tension				
Muscle endurance: sustaining muscle contraction				
Movement Functions				
Motor reflexes: involuntary reflexes–involuntary contractions of muscles automatically induced by stretching				
Involuntary movement reactions: postural, body adjustment, and supporting reactions				
Control of voluntary movement: eye-hand and eye-foot coordination, bilateral integration, crossing midline, fine and gross motor control, oculomotor control				
Gait patterns: movements used to walk				

(continued)

ACTIVITY 6-7 (CONTINUED)

FUNCTION	NONE	MINIMALLY CHALLENGED	GREATLY CHALLENGED	HOW IT IS USED
Cardiovascular, Hematological, Immunological, and Respiratory Systems Functions				
Cardiovascular system: blood pressure, heart rate and rhythm				
Hematological and immunological systems				
Respiratory system: rate, rhythm, and depth of respiration				
Additional functions of the cardiovascular and respiratory systems: physical endurance, stamina, aerobic capacity				
Voice and Speech; Digestive, Metabolic, and Endocrine Systems; and Genitourinary and Reproductive Systems Functions				
Voice and speech: rhythm and fluency, alternative vocalization functions				
Digestive, metabolic, and endocrine systems				
Genitourinary and reproductive systems: urinary, genital, and reproductive functions				
Skin and Related Structures Functions				
Skin: protection, repair				
Hair and nails				

REFERENCES

Al-Hilawani, Y. (2003). Measuring students' metacognition in real life situations. *American Annals of the Deaf, 148*(3), 233-242.

Al-Hilawani, Y., Easterbrooks, S., & Marchant, G. (2002). Metacognitive ability from a theory of mind perspective: A cross-cultural study of students with and without hearing loss. *American Annals of the Deaf, 147,* 38-47.

American Occupational Therapy Association. (2014). Occupational therapy practice framework: Domain and process (3rd ed.). *American Journal of Occupational Therapy, 68*(Suppl. 1), S1-S48. Retrieved from http://dx.doi.org/10.5014/ajot.2014.682006.

Barco, P., Grosson, B., Bolesta, M., Werts, D., & Stout, R. (1991). *Cognitive rehabilitation for persons with traumatic brain injury.* Baltimore, MD: Paul H. Brooks Publishing.

Barnard, C. (1995). Mind in everyday affairs: An examination into logical and non-logical thought processes. *Journal of Management History, 1,* 7-28.

Bolding, D., Adler, C., Tipton-Burton, M., & Lillie, S. (2009). Mobility. In E. Crepeau, E. Cohn, & B. Boyt Schell (Eds.), *Willard and Spackman's occupational therapy* (11th ed., pp. 195-247). Philadelphia, PA: Lippincott Williams & Wilkins.

Breines, E. (2009). Therapeutic occupations and modalities. In H. Pendleton & W. Schultz-Krohn (Eds.), *Pedretti's occupational therapy: Practice skills for physical dysfunction* (pp. 658-679). St. Louis, MO: Mosby Elsevier.

Brown, A. (1978). Knowing when, where, and how to remember: A problem of metacognition. In R. Glaser (Ed.), *Advances in instructional psychology* (pp. 55-113). Hillsdale, NJ: Erlbaum.

Buckley, K., & Poole, S. (2004). Activity analysis. In H. Hinojosa & M. Blount (Eds.), *The texture of life* (pp. 69-114). Bethesda, MD: AOTA Press.

Bukowski, E. (2000). *Muscular analysis of everyday activities.* Thorofare, NJ: SLACK Incorporated.

Chang, E. & Ro, T. (2007). Maintenance of the visual stability in the human posterior parietal cortex. *Journal of Cognitive Neuroscience, 19*(2), 266-274.

Cooper, C., & Abrams, M. (2006). Evaluation of sensation and intervention for sensory dysfunction. In H. Pendleton & W. Schultz-Krohn (Eds.), *Pedretti's occupational therapy: Practice skills for physical dysfunction* (pp. 513-531). St. Louis, MO: Mosby Elsevier.

Crosson, C., Barco, P., Velozo, C., Bolesta, M., Cooper, P., & Werts, D. (1989). Awareness and compensation in post-acute head injury rehabilitation. *Journal of Clinical and Experimental Neuropsychology, 2,* 355-363.

de Bruin, A. (2008). Evaluation of vestibular proprioceptive (VPP) functioning in children: Identification of relevant test items. *South African Journal of Occupational Therapy, 38*(3), 14-17.

Dunn, W. (2009). Sensation and sensory processing. In E. Crepeau, E. Cohn, & B. Boyt Schell (Eds.), *Willard and Spackman's occupational therapy* (11th ed., pp. 777-791). Philadelphia, PA: Lippincott Williams & Wilkins.

Flavell, J. (1979). Metacognition and cognitive monitoring: A new era in psychological inquiry. *American Psychologist, 34,* 906-911.

Levy, L. (2005). Cognitive aging in perspective: Information processing, cognition and memory. In N. Katz (Ed.), *Cognition and occupation across the life span* (2nd ed., pp. 305-325). Bethesda, MD: American Occupational Therapy Association.

Mosby's dictionary of medicine, nursing & health professions. (2006). St. Louis, MO: Mosby Elsevier.

Munguba, M., Valdes, M., & Da Silva, C. (2008). The application of an occupational therapy nutrition education programme for children who are obese. *Occupational Therapy International, 15*(1), 56-70.

Parente, R., & Anderson, J. (1991). *Retraining memory: Techniques and applications.* Houston, TX: CSY Publishing.

Parker, R. (1990). *Traumatic brain injury and neuropsychological impairment.* New York, NY: Springer-Verlag.

Preston, L. (2009). Evaluation of motor control. In H. Pendleton & W. Schultz-Krohn (Eds.), *Pedretti's occupational therapy: Practice skills for physical dysfunction* (pp. 403-428). St. Louis, MO: Mosby Elsevier.

Stedman's medical dictionary for the health professions and nursing (7th ed). (2012). Philadephia, PA: Lippincott Williams & Wilkins.

Warren, M. (2009). Evaluation and treatment of visual deficits following brain injury. In E. Crepeau, E. Cohn, & B. Boyt Schell (Eds.), *Willard and Spackman's occupational therapy* (11th ed., pp. 532-572). Philadelphia, PA: Lippincott Williams & Wilkins.

White, B. (2009). Psychobiological factors. In E. Crepeau, E. Cohn, & B. Boyt Schell (Eds.), *Willard and Spackman's occupational therapy* (11th ed., pp. 716-738). Philadelphia, PA: Lippincott Williams & Wilkins.

World Health Organization. (2001). *International classification of functioning, disability, and health.* Geneva, Switzerland: Author.

Zemke, R. (1994). Task skills, problem solving, and social interaction. In C. B. Royeen (Ed.), *AOTA self study series: Cognitive rehabilitation.* Bethesda, MD: American Occupational Therapy Association.

Zoltan, B. (2007). *Vision, perception, and cognition* (4th ed.). Thorofare, NJ: SLACK Incorporated.

STEPS TO ACTIVITY ANALYSIS

Step 1: Determine What Is Being Analyzed
Chapter 2

Step 2: Determine the Relevance and Importance to the Client
Chapter 3

Step 3: Determine the Sequence and Timing
Chapter 4

Step 4: Determine Object, Space, and Social Demands
Chapter 5

Step 5: Determine Required Body Functions
Chapter 6

Step 6: Determine Required Body Structures
Chapter 7

Step 7: Determine Required Actions and Performance Skills
Chapter 8

7

Step 6: Determine Required Body Structures

OBJECTIVES

- Define *body structures* according to the *Framework*.
- Identify the steps to determining the body structures required of an activity.
- Understand why OT practitioners need to have a basic understanding of how body structures influence performance in activities.
- Define the body structures included in the eyes and ears, voice and speech systems, and the cardiovascular, immune, respiratory, digestive, metabolic, endocrine, genitourinary, and reproductive systems, as well as movement and skin-related structures.
- Identify the body functions influenced by each specific body structure.
- Understand how body systems work collaboratively to meet the demands of activities.

Body structures are those anatomical parts that support body functions (AOTA, 2014). This includes the limbs, organs, and structures of each organ. For example, to allow a person to use his or her respiratory

functions to breathe at the needed rate, the structure of the lungs and circulatory system must work efficiently and be intact. Each of the body functions listed in the *Framework* is supported by one or more body structure systems. The *Framework* utilizes the classification of body systems which is used by the WHO in the ICF. There are eight broad categories, some of which include several systems categorized together.

Instead of defining each of the body structures, the *Framework* refers the reader to the ICF classifications and states:

> Occupational therapy practitioners have knowledge of body structures and understand broadly the interaction that occurs between these structures to support health and participation in life through engagement in occupation. Some therapists may specialize in evaluating and intervening with a specific structure as it is related to supporting performance and engagement in occupations and activities targeted for intervention. (AOTA, 2008, p. 637)

It is assumed that, through entry-level OT education, the clinician will gain a basic understanding of

Thomas H.
Occupation-Based Activity Analysis, Second Edition (pp 135-153).
© 2015 SLACK Incorporated.

the different body systems and how they support daily activities. The structures of body systems influence body functions and are thus involved in the requirements for activity. Part of analyzing an activity is understanding which body systems are required of the activity being analyzed. Identifying the extent to which each body *function* is utilized, which you learned how to do in the last chapter, will help in determining which body structures are required of an activity. Body structures support body functions; thus, by identifying the functions, you will be able to identify the needed structures. For example, by looking at the list of body functions required for washing one's hair in the shower, we will see that the sensation of touch is used to feel the soapsuds and where the hair is as it is being washed. The touch receptors in the tips of the fingers receive information from what is being touched and send an electrical signal along nerves that run up the arm to the spinal cord and then from the spinal cord to the brain. In the brain, the signal is interpreted. All of these anatomical structures are required in order to sense what is being touched. The lack of a particular structure or damage to a part of the structure can cause deficiencies in functioning. As we examine the different body structure systems, the body functions that rely on them will be identified and the connections between them will become more evident.

While identifying the body functions required for particular activities is a good way to begin, some structures are required for an activity even though they do not support a body function. This is true when a particular part of the body interacts with elements of the environment or actions that occur or is used in conjunction with objects used in the activity. An example of this is the cranial bones, which are part of the structures related to movement. These are the bones that enclose the brain, making up the skull. These hard bones serve to protect the brain from impacts due to external forces. These bones will be very necessary when a person is engaging in occupations in which the head comes into contact with an object, such as a soccer ball when playing soccer. Another example is when the eyelids and eyebrows are used in communicating (i.e., winking or raising the eyebrows in expressions of emotion). So in analyzing an activity for the needed body structures, think about which body parts are used during the activity, as well as the body functions that need support from body structures.

Here are some steps to identifying required body structures:

- Match the body functions that are needed with the supporting body structures.
- Identify which body parts are used during the activity.
- Determine which parts of the body come in contact with external forces.

The following sections give a brief description of each of the body structure systems identified by the *Framework* along with the ICF definition of the structures that make up that system. Each of the listed structures has corresponding body functions that it supports. While this presents an introduction to each of the systems as it relates to engagement in occupations, further reading is recommended for a more in-depth understanding of particular body systems.

STRUCTURES OF THE NERVOUS SYSTEM

The brain is the central structure of the nervous system, both processing sensory information and sending motor responses. It is the brain and its corresponding structures that control all thought processes. The function of the nervous system and each of its structures is complex; volumes of texts and courses are dedicated to this subject. The following is a brief introduction to the basic functions of each of the structures.

The structures of the brain include the lobes of the brain, midbrain, cerebellum, brainstem, and cranial nerves. The brain has four lobes: occipital, temporal, frontal, and parietal. The primary function of the occipital lobe is to process visual information. The temporal lobe controls learning, memory, language, and auditory information. The frontal lobe is involved in movement, judgment, emotional behavior, problem solving, and language expression. The parietal lobe controls the processing of visuospatial and somatosensory (sensations from the body) information, as well as the interpretation of language. The midbrain, or mesencephalon, is a relay center for visual and auditory information and controls movements of the eyes and body (*Mosby's Dictionary of Medicine*, 2006). The diencephalon—comprising the thalamus, hypothalamus, subthalamus, and epithalamus—is a small but essential hub for many functions of the brain. It plays a role in sleep, sensation, movement, cognition, emotion, and arousal. It also serves as a relay station to the brain for data received from the sensory systems. The hypothalamus, which is part of the diencephalon, controls autonomic, endocrine, and emotional functions (Filley, 2002). The basal ganglia control the subconscious modulation of movements, especially organizing movements so as to prevent tremors ("Basal ganglia," 2002). When this area of the brain is impaired, as in Parkinson's disease, muscular tremors become uncontrollable. The cerebellum is primarily responsible for coordination, postural control, equilibrium, and muscle tone ("Cerebellum," 2002).

The brainstem controls many essential body functions. This includes sleep/wake cycles, consciousness, pupillary size, voluntary and involuntary movements of the eyes, body movement, posture, touch, temperature, pain, hearing, movement against gravity, taste, salivation, chewing and swallowing, gastrointestinal functions, urination, breathing, blood flow/pressure, and cardiac functions ("Functions," 2002). There are 12 cranial nerves, which provide sensory and motor neural transmission for the head and neck. Structurally, these nerves are connected to the brain and are thus considered structures of the brain. Each of the cranial nerves sends and receives messages for specific functions, including smell, vision, eye movement, sensations of the head and face, chewing, hearing, balance, movement of the tongue, taste, and swallowing functions ("Cranial nerves," 2002). Table 7-1 describes which body functions are reliant on each of the different structures of the brain.

The structures of the spinal cord also serve a purpose in the nervous system as relays for sensory and motor signals. The spinal cord contains nerves that travel from the base of the brain through the spinal column (which is protected by bony vertebrae) and down to the bottom of the spinal column. The spinal cord works as a conduit for messages being sent to and from the body. Structures within the spinal cord also control reflexive actions, bypassing the brain. Thirty-one pairs of spinal nerves branch out from the spinal cord, each pair emerging from one of the 31 vertebrae. These nerves extend out to all areas of the body (*The Human Body Book*, 2009). The spinal nerves that emerge at each level of vertebrae control and send neural impulses from a different area of the body. Each set of spinal nerves is named according to the level of the vertebral column from which

they emerge. Thus, there are 8 cervical, 12 thoracic, 5 lumbar, and 5 sacral pairs and 1 coccygeal pair. Each pair has posterior roots that are primarily sensory neurons and ventral (anterior) roots that contain motor neurons (*Mosby's Dictionary of Medicine*, 2006). These spinal nerves control sensation and motor movement.

The meninges are the three membranes that encompass and protect the spinal cord and brain. The sympathetic nervous system automatically prepares the body for emergency or stressful situations, while the parasympathetic nervous systems works to restore the body to a more relaxed state. In the face of danger or stress, the sympathetic nervous system causes the pupils to dilate, the bronchial tubes to open, the heart rate to increase, and the stomach's digestive functions to slow. As the danger or stressor is removed, the parasympathetic nervous system constricts the pupils and bronchial tubes, decreases the heart rate, and restores normal digestion (*The Human Body Book*, 2009) (see Table 7-1).

EYES, EARS, AND RELATED STRUCTURES

The structures of the eye are those that allow visual data to be sent to the brain for interpretation. Without intact structures within and around the eye, images may be distorted or not interpretable. This includes the structures that make up the eyeball itself, as well as the structures that surround it and contribute to sight. The same is true of the ear and the structures that allow for hearing. There are external, middle, and inner ear structures that work in conjunction with each other to allow for the reception of sounds, as well as the determination of the body's position in space (Table 7-2).

STRUCTURES INVOLVED IN VOICE AND SPEECH

Several parts of the body control the ability to speak. Typically, the larynx is thought of as the primary structure involved in speech, but in order to form words and project the sounds, the structures of the nose, mouth, and pharynx are also required. The

TABLE 7-1
BODY STRUCTURES OF THE NERVOUS SYSTEM

BODY STRUCTURE	BODY FUNCTIONS RELIANT ON THIS STRUCTURE	
Frontal lobe	Judgment	Appropriate thought content
	Concept formation	Execution of learned movement patterns
	Metacognition	
	Cognitive flexibility	Coping and behavioral regulation
	Insight	Emotional stability
	Attention	Motivation
	Awareness	Impulse control
	Sustained, selective, and divided attention	Body image
		Self-concept
	Memory	Self-esteem
	Temporal relationships	Orientation
	Recognition	Eye-hand/foot coordination
	Categorization	Bilateral integration
	Generalization	Crossing midline
	Awareness of reality	Fine and gross motor control
	Logical/coherent thought	Walking patterns
Temporal lobe	Concept formation	Execution of learned movement patterns
	Memory	
	Discrimination of sensations (auditory)	Coping and behavioral regulation
	Recognition	Orientation
	Categorization	Tolerance of ambient sounds
	Generalization	Awareness of location and distance of sounds
Parietal lobe	Spatial relationships	Touch
	Discrimination of sensations (visual)	Pain
	Awareness of body position and space	Thermal awareness
	Taste	
Occipital lobe	Detection/registration	Visual awareness of environment at various distances
	Modulation	
Midbrain (mesencephalon)	Discrimination of senses (auditory, visual)	Awareness of location and distance of sounds
	Execution of learned movement patterns	Eye-hand/eye-foot coordination
		Crossing midline
	Detection/registration	Fine and gross motor control
	Modulation	Oculomotor control
	Visual awareness at various distance	Walking patterns
	Tolerance of ambient sounds	

(continued)

TABLE 7-1 (CONTINUED)
BODY STRUCTURES OF THE NERVOUS SYSTEM

BODY STRUCTURE	BODY FUNCTIONS RELIANT ON THIS STRUCTURE	
Diencephalon	Judgment	Modulation
	Concept formation	Integration of sensations from the body and environment
	Metacognition	Tolerance of ambient sounds
	Cognitive flexibility	Awareness of location and distance of sounds
	Insight	
	Attention	Sensation of securely moving against gravity
	Awareness	
	Coping and behavioral regulation	Taste
	Body image	Smell
	Self-concept	Proprioception
	Self-esteem	Touch
	Execution of learned movement patterns	Thermal awareness
		Eye-hand/foot coordination
	Arousal, consciousness	Bilateral integration
	Orientation	Crossing midline
	Sleep	Fine and gross motor control
	Discrimination of senses (auditory, tactile, visual, olfactory, gustatory, vestibular-proprioceptive)	Walking patterns
		Blood pressure functions
	Multisensory processing	Endocrine system functions
Basal ganglia	Eye-hand/eye-foot coordination	Fine and gross motor control
	Bilateral integration	Walking patterns
	Crossing midline	
Cerebellum	Eye-hand/eye-foot coordination	Muscle tone
	Crossing midline	Walking patterns
	Fine and gross motor control	Sensation of moving securely against gravity
	Righting and supporting	
Brainstem	Arousal	Oculomotor control
	Consciousness	Righting and supporting
	Sleep	Eye-hand/eye-foot coordination
	Modulation	Bilateral integration
	Visual awareness at various distances	Crossing the midline
	Sensations of securely moving against gravity	Fine and gross motor control
		Walking patterns
	Touch	Blood pressure functions
	Pain	Cardiovascular system functions

(continued)

TABLE 7-1 (CONTINUED)
BODY STRUCTURES OF THE NERVOUS SYSTEM

BODY STRUCTURE	BODY FUNCTIONS RELIANT ON THIS STRUCTURE	
Brainstem (continued)	Thermal awareness Tolerance of ambient sounds Awareness of location and distance of sounds	Respiratory functions Digestive system functions Urinary functions
Cranial nerves	Detection/registration Modulation Visual awareness of environment and various distances Awareness of location and distance of sounds Sensation of securely moving against gravity	Taste Smell Awareness of body position and space Touch Fine and gross motor coordination Oculomotor control Digestive system functions
Spinal cord	Awareness of body position and space Touch Pain Thermal awareness Muscle tone Asymmetrical and symmetrical tonic neck reflex Righting and supporting Eye-hand/foot coordination	Bilateral coordination Crossing midline Fine and gross motor control Walking patterns Blood pressure functions Heart rate Voice functions Digestive system functions Urinary functions Genital and reproductive functions
Spinal nerves	Awareness of body position and space Touch Pain Thermal awareness Muscle tone Asymmetrical and symmetrical tonic neck reflex Righting and supporting Eye-hand/foot coordination	Bilateral coordination Crossing midline Fine and gross motor control Walking patterns Blood pressure functions Heart rate Voice functions Digestive system functions Urinary functions Genital and reproductive functions
Meninges	Judgment Concept formation Metacognition Cognitive flexibility Insight	Self-concept Self-esteem Orientation Detection/registration Modulation

(continued)

TABLE 7-1 (CONTINUED)
BODY STRUCTURES OF THE NERVOUS SYSTEM

BODY STRUCTURE	BODY FUNCTIONS RELIANT ON THIS STRUCTURE	
Meninges (continued)	Attention Awareness Sustained, selective, and divided attention Memory Discrimination of sensations Multisensory processing Sensory memory Spatial relationships Temporal relationships Recognition Categorization Generalization Awareness of reality Logical/coherent thought Appropriate thought content Execution of learned movement patterns Coping and behavioral regulation Emotional stability Motivation Impulse control Body image	Integration of sensations from the body and environment Visual awareness of environment at various distances Tolerance of ambient sounds Awareness of location and distance of sounds Sensation of securely moving against gravity Awareness of body position and space Localizing pain Thermal awareness Muscle tone Asymmetrical tonic neck reflex Symmetrical tonic neck reflex Righting and supporting Eye-hand/foot coordination Bilateral integration Crossing midline Fine and gross motor control Oculomotor control Walking patterns
Sympathetic nervous system	Detection/registration Modulation Integration of sensations from body and environment Visual awareness of environment at various distances	Blood pressure functions Rate, rhythm, and depth of respiration Digestive system function
Parasympathetic nervous system	Detection/registration Modulation Integration of sensations from body and environment Visual awareness of environment at various distances	Blood pressure functions Rate, rhythm, and depth of respiration Digestive system function

TABLE 7-2
EYES, EARS, AND RELATED STRUCTURES

BODY STRUCTURE	BODY FUNCTIONS RELIANT ON THIS STRUCTURE	
Eyeball: Conjunctiva, cornea, iris, retina, lens, vitreous body	Visual Eye-hand/eye-foot coordination	
Structures around eye: Lacrimal gland, eyelid, eyebrow, external ocular muscles	Visual Control of voluntary movement	
Structure of external ear	Hearing	
Structures of middle ear: Tympanic membrane, eustachian canal, ossicles	Hearing	
Structures of inner ear: Cochlea, vestibular labyrinth, semicircular canals, internal auditory meatus	Hearing Vestibular	Involuntary movement reactions Gait patterns

body functions reliant on these structures are only the voice and speech functions (Table 7-3).

STRUCTURES OF THE CARDIOVASCULAR, IMMUNOLOGICAL, AND RESPIRATORY SYSTEMS

The ICF and the *Framework* lump these three major body systems together. While each of them serves a very specific function, all of them are essential to maintaining human life. The next set of body structures and related body functions are considered separately, so that it is evident what each of them provides (Tables 7-4 to 7-7). Each of these systems is reliant on the others and contributes to the existence and survival of other systems. For example, without adequate circulation, the neurological systems would be ineffective. The circulatory, respiratory and immunological systems are required to sustain human life. However, when doing an activity analysis, do not consider what is required to sustain life, but what is challenged because of the activity demands. For example, the respiratory system is needed to sustain life, but it is challenged when engaged in the activity of blowing bubbles. In analyzing an activity for the body system

requirements in this area, think about which body functions are challenged and which, in turn, challenge the corresponding body structures.

Cardiovascular System

The heart's atria and ventricles serve to pump blood to the lungs, where the blood takes up oxygen; the oxygenated blood is then pumped throughout the body. The heart performs this action an average of 70 times per minute. It receives deoxygenated blood from the body via the veins. The veins deliver blood from tissues throughout the body to the heart to be reoxygenated. Once the blood has been passed through the lungs, it is sent out to the tissues of the body via arteries (*Mosby's Dictionary of Medicine*, 2006). Capillaries form networks of thin-walled blood vessels where oxygenated blood from the arteries is delivered to the body and then returned to the heart via the veins. Capillaries exist throughout the body, providing oxygen and other nutrients to the tissues ("Capillaries," 2000) (see Table 7-4).

Immunological System

The immune system functions to protect the body against infection and disease. The body protects itself

TABLE 7-3
STRUCTURES INVOLVED IN VOICE AND SPEECH FUNCTIONS

BODY STRUCTURE	BODY FUNCTIONS RELIANT ON THIS STRUCTURE
Structures of the nose: External nose, nasal septum, nasal fossae	Voice and speech functions
Structure of the mouth: Teeth, gums, hard palate, soft palate, tongue, lips	Voice and speech functions
Structure of pharynx: Nasal pharynx and oral pharynx	Voice and speech functions Vocalization
Structure of larynx: Vocal folds	Voice and speech functions

TABLE 7-4
BODY STRUCTURES OF THE CARDIOVASCULAR SYSTEM

BODY STRUCTURE	BODY FUNCTIONS RELIANT ON THIS STRUCTURE	
Heart: Atria, ventricles	Consciousness Cardiovascular system functions	Physical endurance Stamina and fatigability
Arteries	Blood pressure Muscle endurance	Physical endurance Stamina and fatigability
Veins	Blood pressure Muscle endurance	Physical endurance Stamina and fatigability
Capillaries	Blood pressure functions	Muscle endurance

TABLE 7-5
BODY STRUCTURES OF THE IMMUNOLOGICAL SYSTEM

BODY STRUCTURE	BODY FUNCTIONS RELIANT ON THIS STRUCTURE	
Lymphatic vessels	Joint mobility Gait patterns	Immunological system Skin functions
Lymphatic nodes	Joint mobility Gait patterns	Immunological system Skin functions
Thymus	Joint mobility Skin functions	Immunological system
Spleen	Skin functions	Immunological system
Bone marrow	Skin functions	Immunological system

TABLE 7-6
BODY STRUCTURES OF THE RESPIRATORY SYSTEM

BODY STRUCTURE	BODY FUNCTIONS RELIANT ON THIS STRUCTURE	
Trachea	Respiratory system functions Physical endurance	Voice functions Aerobic capacity
Lungs: Bronchial tree, alveoli	Respiratory system functions Stamina Voice functions	Fatigability Physical endurance Aerobic capacity
Thoracic cage	Respiratory system functions Stamina Voice functions	Fatigability Physical endurance Aerobic capacity
Muscles of respiration: Intercostal muscles, diaphragm	Respiratory system functions Stamina Voice functions	Fatigability Physical endurance Aerobic capacity

TABLE 7-7
STRUCTURES OF THE DIGESTIVE, METABOLIC, AND ENDOCRINE SYSTEMS

BODY STRUCTURE	BODY FUNCTIONS RELIANT ON THIS STRUCTURE	
Salivary glands	Digestive system functions	Taste
Esophagus	Digestive system functions	
Stomach	Digestive system functions	Metabolic system
Intestines: Small and large	Digestive system functions	Metabolic system
Pancreas	Digestive system functions	Metabolic system
Liver	Digestive system functions Metabolic system	Immunological system functions Endocrine system
Gallbladder and ducts	Digestive system functions	Metabolic system
Endocrine glands: Pituitary, thyroid, parathyroid, adrenal	Genital and reproductive functions Hair and nail functions Metabolic system functions	Digestive system functions Emotional Endocrine system functions Appetite

through an elaborate system that includes the thymus, bone marrow, lymph tissues, lymph nodes, spleen, and lymph vessels (*Mosby's Dictionary of Medicine*, 2006). The thymus is a lymph gland located near the sternum; it is the primary site for the creation of T cells. T cells originate in the bone marrow but are sent to the thymus to mature, after which they travel to other lymph tissues in the body to fight off antigens or foreign substances (*Taber's Cyclopedic Medical Dictionary*, 2001). Lymph nodes are small kidney-shaped collections of tissue from which lymph fluid flows. Antibodies are produced in the lymph nodes and then travel to the blood via the lymph fluid. Lymph nodes are located throughout the body, either singly or in clusters along the lymphatic vessels, which run from the head, down the neck, and into the arms, through the trunk, and down the legs (*Taber's Cyclopedic Medical Dictionary*, 2001). The spleen is also essential to the immune system in that it creates lymphocytes and antibodies to help fight off invaders. The spleen also works to remove cell debris, old or damaged cells, and cells that are coated with antibodies (*Taber's Cyclopedic Medical Dictionary*, 2001). It is located in the upper left quadrant of the abdomen, near the stomach (see Table 7-5).

Respiratory System

The respiratory system structures serve to bring oxygen into the body via the blood. This occurs by inhalation, which is controlled by movement of the intercostal muscles surrounding the rib cage, as well as by the diaphragm. When the diaphragm contracts, it flattens itself downward, away from the lungs, creating pressure that allows the lungs to expand. When the lungs are allowed to expand, air is pulled in through the trachea, a tube made of cartilage that extends from the larynx down to two branches, one to each lung. The thoracic cage, which consists of the 12 pairs of rib bones, the sternum, and the thoracic vertebrae, which run up the back of the cage, protects and surrounds the lungs and heart. The thoracic cage moves along with inspiration and expiration and provides the structure needed for negative and positive airway pressure, which pulls air in and out with each contraction and relaxation of the diaphragm (see Table 7-6).

STRUCTURES RELATED TO THE DIGESTIVE, METABOLIC, AND ENDOCRINE SYSTEMS

The digestive, metabolic, and endocrine systems work together to effectively utilize food as an energy source. The digestive system begins its work as food enters the mouth and the salivary glands produce saliva to begin breaking down food particles. As food is swallowed, it travels down the esophagus to the stomach, where the digestive process begins. Protein digestion begins in the stomach, but most absorption of food occurs in the small intestine. The stomach does absorb liquids, however. Food travels from the stomach to the small intestine, where it is joined by bile from the liver and gallbladder and pancreatic juice from the pancreas. It is in the small intestine that essential nutrients and fluids are absorbed into the blood, which is then sent to the liver. The liver has multiple functions related to metabolizing food molecules. The liver also detoxifies the bloodstream by breaking down harmful substances, such as alcohol or drugs. Hemoglobin by-products are broken down and sent out into the feces to be eliminated. The liver produces protein and clotting factors; it also stores copper, iron, and vitamins B_{12}, A, D, E, and K (*Taber's Cyclopedic Medical Dictionary*, 2001). Endocrine glands excrete hormones directly into the bloodstream. The pituitary, thyroid, parathyroid, and adrenal glands all contribute to metabolic activities (the utilization of food and water that are put into the body), as well as growth and sexual development (see Table 7-7).

STRUCTURES RELATED TO THE GENITOURINARY AND REPRODUCTIVE SYSTEMS

The structures of the genitourinary system relate to all structures that allow for urination and reproduction. In men, many of the structures for urination and for reproduction are shared; in women, most of the structures are separate. The urinary system comprises the kidneys, which serve to filter the blood and eliminate wastes through the urine. The urine that is created in the kidneys is sent to the bladder via the ureter, which is a tube that runs from each kidney into the bladder. From the bladder, the urine passes through the urethra out of the body. The pelvic floor comprises muscles and ligaments that hold the pelvic organs, which include the muscles required for urination, as well as those needed to support the reproductive organs. A failure in the functioning of the pelvic floor is one of the leading causes of urinary incontinence (*Mosby's Dictionary of Medicine*, 2006). Structures of the female reproductive system include the ovaries, uterus, breasts, nipples, and external genitalia; the male reproductive system includes the testes, penis, and prostate. The male relies on the structures of the penis and prostate for urination as well (Table 7-8).

TABLE 7-8 STRUCTURES OF THE GENITOURINARY AND REPRODUCTIVE SYSTEMS	
BODY STRUCTURE	**BODY FUNCTIONS RELIANT ON THIS STRUCTURE**
Urinary system: Kidneys, ureters, bladder, urethra	Urinary functions
Structure of pelvic floor	Reproductive functions Walking patterns
Structure of reproductive system: Ovaries, uterus, breast and nipple, vagina and external genitalia, testes, penis, prostate	Reproductive functions

STRUCTURES RELATED TO MOVEMENT

Of all of the body structure categories, this one involves the greatest number of related structures. In analyzing an activity that requires movement, it will be important to identify the specific body structures required for the task. For this reason, the ICF details very specific muscular and joint structures throughout the body. Determining which of these structures is needed for an activity will require an examination of each of the steps and specific movements required of each body part (Table 7-9).

SKIN AND RELATED STRUCTURES

The structures related to skin and hair are part of many grooming and bathing activities, such as washing hair and trimming nails. Thus, these body structures would be required of those occupations. Without hair, the task of washing one's hair becomes unneeded. Thus, for this body structure category, it easier to think of the occupations or activities for which hair, skin, and nails are required instead of thinking of what body functions are reliant on these structures (Table 7-10).

CONCLUSION

Body structures are those physical aspects of organs, limbs, and structures of each organ that support body functioning. Structures work together to keep the human body healthy and allow for participation in daily activities. The extent to which each body structure is challenged relies on the demands of the activities (the steps, space, objects, and social demands) and is linked to the body functions utilized. It is important for OT practitioners to recognize the importance of each of the body systems and how each one can influence performance of activities. The body systems work collaboratively and are often not solely responsible for a single function. For example, many of our mental functions rely not only on the structures on the nervous system, but also on the cardiovascular system's ability to deliver oxygen-rich blood to the brain. While this chapter offers a brief introduction to the primary functions of each body system, the body is much more complex and further investigation into a specific system is warranted for specialization.

QUESTIONS

1. Washing one's hair in the shower challenges which body structures (beyond what is required to sustain life)?
2. Why is it necessary to know which body structures are required for an activity?
3. How do you determine which body structures are necessary for an activity?
4. What are the structures of the nervous system? What are at least 10 body functions the nervous system structures support?
5. What body functions do the lymph structures support?
6. Voice functions are supported by which body structures?

TABLE 7-9
BODY STRUCTURES RELATED TO MOVEMENT

BODY STRUCTURE	BODY FUNCTIONS RELIANT ON THIS STRUCTURE	
Bones of cranium	None	
Bones of face	Digestive system functions	
Bones of neck region	Motor reflexes	Involuntary movement reactions
Joints of head and neck	Digestive system functions Joint mobility	Motor reflexes
Bones of shoulder region	Motor reflexes	Involuntary movement reactions
Joints of shoulder region	Joint mobility Joint stability	Motor reflexes Involuntary movement reactions
Muscles of shoulder region	Muscle power (shoulder) Muscle endurance	Motor reflexes Involuntary movement reactions
Bones of upper arm	Motor reflexes	Involuntary movement reactions
Elbow joint	Joint mobility (elbow) Joint stability	Motor reflexes Involuntary movement reactions
Muscles of upper arm	Muscle power	Motor reflexes
Ligaments and fascia of upper arm	Joint mobility (upper arm)	
Bones of forearm	Motor reflexes	
Wrist joint	Joint mobility (wrist) Joint stability	Motor reflexes Involuntary movement reactions
Muscles of forearm	Muscle power	Motor reflexes
Ligaments and fascia of forearm	Joint mobility (forearm)	Joint stability
Muscles of hand	Motor reflexes Control of voluntary movement	Involuntary movement reactions
Ligaments and fascia of hand	Joint mobility	Joint stability
Bones of pelvic region	Motor reflexes	Involuntary movement reactions
Joints of pelvic region	Joint mobility Joint stability	Motor reflexes Involuntary movement reactions
Muscles of pelvic region	Motor reflexes Genitourinary and reproductive system	Involuntary movement reactions
Ligaments and fascia of pelvic region	Joint mobility Joint stability	Motor reflexes Involuntary movement reactions
Bones of thigh	Motor reflexes	Involuntary movement reactions
Hip joint	Joint mobility Joint stability	Motor reflexes Involuntary movement reactions

(continued)

TABLE 7-9 (CONTINUED)
BODY STRUCTURES RELATED TO MOVEMENT

BODY STRUCTURE	BODY FUNCTIONS RELIANT ON THIS STRUCTURE	
Muscles of thigh	Motor reflexes	Involuntary movement reactions
Ligaments and fascia of thigh	Joint mobility	Motor reflexes
	Joint stability	Involuntary movement reactions
Bones of lower leg	Motor reflexes	Involuntary movement reactions
Knee joint	Joint mobility	Joint stability
Muscles of lower leg	Motor reflexes	Involuntary movement reactions
Ligaments and fascia of lower leg	Joint mobility	Motor reflexes
	Joint stability	Involuntary movement reactions
Bones of ankle and foot	Motor reflexes	Involuntary movement reactions
Ankle, foot, and toe joints	Joint mobility	Righting and supporting
	Joint stability	
Muscle of ankle and foot	Motor reflexes	Involuntary movement reactions
Ligaments and fascia of ankle and foot	Joint mobility	Motor reflexes
	Joint stability	Involuntary movement reactions
Cervical vertebral column	Joint mobility	Joint stability
Lumbar vertebral column	Joint mobility	Joint stability
Sacral vertebral column	Joint mobility	Joint stability
Muscles of trunk	Motor reflexes	Involuntary movement reactions
Ligaments and fascia of trunk	Joint mobility	Joint stability

TABLE 7-10
SKIN AND RELATED STRUCTURES

BODY STRUCTURE	BODY FUNCTIONS RELIANT ON THIS STRUCTURE	
Areas of skin: Head, neck, shoulder, upper extremity, pelvic region, lower extremities, trunk and back	Joint mobility Pain Skin functions	Touch Sensitivity to temperature and pressure
Structure of skin glands: Sweat and sebaceous	Skin functions	
Structure of nails: Fingernails, toenails	Hair and nail functions	
Structure of hair	Hair and nail functions	

ACTIVITIES

1. Continue to analyze the activity of washing hair in the shower by completing Activity 7-1.
2. Body structure charades: Write each of the following body structures on a piece of paper and place the papers in a hat or bowl:
   - Frontal lobe
   - Temporal lobe
   - Parietal lobe
   - Occipital lobe
   - Eyeball: conjunctiva, cornea, iris, retina, lens, vitreous body
   - Structures around eye: lacrimal gland, eyelid, eyebrow, external ocular muscles
   - Structure of external ear
   - Structure of middle ear: tympanic membrane, eustachian canal, ossicles
   - Structures of inner ear: cochlea, vestibular labyrinth, semicircular canals, internal auditory meatus
   - Structures of the nose: external nose, nasal septum, nasal fossae
   - Structure of the mouth: teeth, gums, hard palate, soft palate, tongue, lips
   - Structure of pharynx: nasal pharynx and oral pharynx
   - Structure of larynx: vocal folds
   - Salivary glands
   - Esophagus
   - Stomach
   - Urinary system: kidneys, ureters, bladder, urethra
   - Structure of reproductive system: ovaries, uterus, breast and nipple, vagina and external genitalia, testes, penis, prostate
   - Bones of cranium
   - Bones of face
   - Bones of neck region
   - Joints of head and neck
   - Bones of shoulder region
   - Joints of shoulder region
   - Muscles of shoulder region
   - Bones of upper arm
   - Elbow joint
   - Muscles of upper arm
   - Ligaments and fascia of upper arm
   - Bones of forearm
   - Wrist joint
   - Muscles of forearm
   - Ligaments and fascia of forearm
   - Bones of hand
   - Joints of hand and fingers
   - Muscles of hand
   - Bones of pelvic region
   - Joints of pelvic region
   - Muscles of pelvic region
   - Bones of thigh
   - Hip joint
   - Muscles of thigh
   - Bones of lower leg
   - Knee joint
   - Muscles of lower leg
   - Bones of ankle and foot
   - Ankle, foot, and toe joints
   - Muscle of ankle and foot
   - Cervical vertebral column
   - Lumbar vertebral column
   - Muscles of trunk
   - Areas of skin: head, neck, shoulder, upper extremity, pelvic region, lower extremities, trunk, back
   - Structure of skin glands: sweat and sebaceous
   - Structure of nails: fingernails, toenails
   - Structure of hair

   Each student will draw one of the body structures and then act out or pantomime an activity in which the body structure is required. The class is to guess which body structure the activity is utilizing.
3. An adaptation of the activity above: Each student draws a body structure from the hat or bowl. Each person is given 1 minute to write down as many activities that he or she can think of that require that body structure. At the 1-minute mark, the students are to pass their papers to the next persons (each student gets his or her neighbor's sheet) and are given 1 minute to think of other activities that have not already been listed.
4. Complete section 10 of the Occupation-Based Activity Analysis form for the occupation that you have been analyzing throughout this book.

ACTIVITY 7-1

Determine what body structures are required in the activity of washing hair in the shower.

CATEGORY	BODY STRUCTURE	REQUIRED? (CHECK IF YES)
Nervous system	Frontal lobe	
	Temporal lobe	
	Parietal lobe	
	Occipital lobe	
	Midbrain	
	Diencephalon	
	Basal ganglia	
	Cerebellum	
	Brain stem	
	Cranial nerves	
	Spinal cord	
	Spinal nerves	
	Meninges	
	Sympathetic nervous system	
	Parasympathetic nervous system	
Eyes, ears, and related structures	Eyeball: Conjunctiva, cornea, iris, retina, lens, vitreous body	
	Structures around eye: Lachrimal gland, eyelid, eyebrow, external ocular muscles	
	Structure of external ear	
	Structure of middle ear: Tympanic membrane, eustachian canal, ossicles	
	Structures of inner ear: Cochlea, vestibular labyrinth, semicircular canals, internal auditory meatus	
Voice and speech structures	Structures of the nose: External nose, nasal septum, nasal fossae	
	Structure of the mouth: Teeth, gums, hard palate, soft palate, tongue, lips	
	Structure of pharynx: Nasal pharynx and oral pharynx	
	Structure of larynx: Vocal folds	

(continued)

ACTIVITY 7-1 (CONTINUED)

CATEGORY	BODY STRUCTURE	REQUIRED? (CHECK IF YES)
Cardiovascular system	Heart: Atria, ventricles	
	Arteries	
	Veins	
	Capillaries	
Immunological system	Lymphatic vessels	
	Lymphatic nodes	
	Thymus	
	Spleen	
	Bone marrow	
Respiratory system	Trachea	
	Lungs: Bronchial tree, alveoli	
	Thoracic cage	
	Muscles of respiration: Intercostal muscles, diaphragm	
Digestive, metabolic, and endocrine systems	Salivary glands	
	Esophagus	
	Stomach	
	Intestines: Small and large	
	Pancreas	
	Liver	
	Gall bladder and ducts	
	Endocrine glands: Pituitary, thyroid, parathyroid, adrenal	
Genitourinary and reproductive systems	Urinary system: Kidneys, ureters, bladder, urethra	
	Structure of pelvic floor	
	Structures of reproductive system: Ovaries, uterus, breast and nipple, vagina and external genitalia, testes, penis, prostate	
Structures related to movement	Bones of cranium	
	Bones of face	
	Bones of neck region	
	Joints of head and neck	
	Bones of shoulder region	
	Joints of shoulder region	

(continued)

Activity 7-1 (continued)

CATEGORY	BODY STRUCTURE	REQUIRED? (CHECK IF YES)
Structures related to movement	Muscles of shoulder region	
	Bones of upper arm	
	Elbow joint	
	Muscles of upper arm	
	Ligaments and fascia of upper arm	
	Bones of forearm	
	Wrist joint	
	Muscles of forearm	
	Ligaments and fascia of forearm	
	Bones of hand	
	Joints of hand and fingers	
	Muscles of hand	
	Ligaments and fascia of hand	
	Bones of pelvic region	
	Joints of pelvic region	
	Muscles of pelvic region	
	Ligaments and fascia of pelvic region	
	Bones of thigh	
	Hip joint	
	Muscles of thigh	
	Ligaments and fascia of thigh	
	Bones of lower leg	
	Knee joint	
	Muscles of lower leg	
	Ligaments and fascia of lower leg	
	Bones of ankle and foot	
	Ankle, foot, and toe joints	
	Muscle of ankle and foot	
	Ligaments of fascia of ankle and foot	
	Cervical vertebral column	
	Lumbar vertebral column	
	Sacral vertebral column	
	Muscles of trunk	
	Ligaments and fascia of trunk	

(continued)

ACTIVITY 7-1 (CONTINUED)

CATEGORY	BODY STRUCTURE	REQUIRED? (CHECK IF YES)
Skin and related structures	Areas of skin: Head, neck, shoulder, upper extremity, pelvic region, lower extremities, trunk, and back	
	Structure of skin glands: Sweat and sebaceous	
	Structure of nails: Fingernails and toenails	
	Structure of hair	

REFERENCES

American Occupational Therapy Association. (2008). Occupational therapy practice framework: Domain and process (2nd ed.). *American Journal of Occupational Therapy, 62*(6), 609-639.

American Occupational Therapy Association. (2014). Occupational therapy practice framework: Domain and process (3rd ed.). *American Journal of Occupational Therapy, 68*(Suppl. 1), S1-S48. Retrived from http://dx.doi.org/10.5014/ajot.2014.682006

Basal ganglia. (2002). In *Encyclopedia of the human brain*. Oxford, United Kingdom: Elsevier Science & Technology.

Brain. (2004). In W. Craighead and C. Nemeroff (Eds.), *The Concise Corsini encyclopedia of psychology and behavioral science*. Hoboken, NJ: Wiley.

Capillaries. (2000). In *The Royal Society of medicine health encyclopedia*. London, United Kingdom: Bloomsbury. Functions regulated in the brain stem. (2002). In *Encyclopedia of the human brain*. Oxford, United Kingdom: Elsevier Science & Technology.

Cerebellum. (2002). In Encyclopedia of the human brain. Oxford, United Kingdom: Elsevier Science & Technology.

Cranial nerves. (2002). In *Encyclopedia of the human brain*. Oxford, United Kingdom: Elsevier Science & Technology.

Filley, C. (2002). Neuroanatomy. In V. Ramachandran (Ed.), *Encyclopedia of the human brain*. San Francisco, CA: Elsevier Science & Technology.

The human body book: An illustrated guide to its structure, function and disorders (2009). London, United Kingdom: Dorling Kindersley Publishing, Inc.

Mosby's dictionary of medicine, nursing & health professions. (2006). St. Louis, MO: Author.

Taber's cyclopedic medical dictionary. (2001). Philadelphia, PA: F. A. Davis Company.

World Health Organization. (2001). *International classification of functioning, disability, and health.* Geneva, Switzerland: Author.

STEPS TO ACTIVITY ANALYSIS

Step 1: Determine What Is Being Analyzed
Chapter 2

**Step 2: Determine the Relevance
and Importance to the Client**
Chapter 3

Step 3: Determine the Sequence and Timing
Chapter 4

**Step 4: Determine Object, Space,
and Social Demands**
Chapter 5

Step 5: Determine Required Body Functions
Chapter 6

Step 6: Determine Required Body Structures
Chapter 7

Step 7: Determine Required Actions and Performance Skills
Chapter 8

8

Step 7: Determine Required Actions and Performance Skills

OBJECTIVES

- Define performance skills and explain how they differ from body functions.
- Understand what can influence performance skills using perspectives from frames of reference and ecological models.
- Show how to determine the skill level required for an activity.
- Identify the elements of motor skills and the body functions influencing these skills.
- Define the elements of process skills and the body functions influencing these skills.
- Identify the different aspects of social interaction skills and the body functions that influence these skills.

The next step in the activity analysis process is determining the required actions or performance skills. Performance skills are defined as "goal-directed actions that are observable as small units of engagement in daily life occupations" (AOTA, 2014, p. S7). Therefore, performance skills are abilities that are demonstrated through actions and have the potential

to be learned and improved over time. Activities or occupations are made up of actions, which are made up of performance skills. Each of these actions (or steps) can require a single skill or a combination of skills. Performance skills are distinguished from body functions in that they are observable. These are the actions that our clients take in order to complete an activity or occupation. In the activity analysis process (outlined in Table 7 of the *Framework*), this step calls for "required actions and performance skills" that are "required by the client as an inherent part of the activity" (AOTA, 2014, p. S32). Each step identified as required to complete an activity will require the person engaging in the activity to perform certain actions, using specific skills. Each action or skill leads to another, linked together to enable successful completion of the activity.

There are three categories of performance skills: motor, process, and social interaction. Each skill category is further defined by specific skills. For example, in the area of motor skills is the skill of coordination. This skill comes into play, for example, when a person "uses two or more body parts together to manipulate, hold, and/or stabilize task objects without evidence of

Thomas H.
Occupation-Based Activity Analysis, Second Edition (pp 155-178).
© 2015 SLACK Incorporated.

fumbling task objects or slipping from one's grasp" (AOTA, 2014, p. S25). To complete this step of activity analysis, the list of specific skills is used to decide what skill is required of the participant in the activity.

Background

The skills listed have been carefully defined in the *Framework*, using terminology from the *Assessment of Motor and Process Skills* (AMPS) (Fisher & Jones, 2001a, 2011b), the *School Version of the Assessment of Motor and Process Skills* (School AMPS) (Fisher, Bruyze, Hume, & Griswold, 2007), and the *Evaluation of Social Interaction* (ESI) (Fisher & Griswold, 2010). The purpose of the AMPS is to evaluate the quality of performance in ADL. During performance of an activity, an evaluator using the AMPS would assess the client's skill level during performance or the small units of action (Fisher & Jones, 2001a, 2001b). Thus the individual actions required to complete the task and the skill with which they are performed are assessed, not just completion of the activity. From the perspective of activity analysis, we are not assessing a client's skill but rather the skill required to complete an activity; we are evaluating the activity, not the client. The list of skills provided in the *Framework* is not an all-inclusive list of performance skills, but is designed to propose a framework for the most common performance skills.

Determining Required Performance Skills

Determining the performance skills required of an activity calls for the examination of each of the steps used to carry out the activity. For example, the first step in making scrambled eggs (from Chapter 4) is to:

> *Pick up the pan by grasping the handle of the pan with one hand and picking it up.*

This step would require both motor and process skills. Grasping the handle of the pan will require the motor skills of *reaches* and *grips* and the process skills of *chooses* and *handles*. Lifting the pan once the handle is grasped required the motor skills of *stabilizes* and *lifts* and the process skills of *initiates* and *handles*. These performance skills may continue to be required throughout the activity or only for this step. It is through careful analysis of each step that we are able to determine the extent to which each skill is required. A skill that is slightly required might be needed but not for the majority of the activity. A skill that is essential to a majority of the steps of the task is one that would be considered greatly challenged or required.

Performance skills are supported by a person's body functions and body structures and therefore contribute to a person's ability to demonstrate the skills required of an activity. Certain client factors or body functions may need to be present in order for a performance skill to be used. With this understanding, the activity analysis process becomes cyclical and can be used for treatment planning (see Chapter 9). To help clarify how the body functions play a role in performance skills, let's again look at the activity of making scrambled eggs. In the first step, we found that the performance skill of *grips* is required to grasp on to the handle of the pan. This performance skill is supported by the body functions of muscle power, joint mobility, and joint stability. Also, the body structures related to movement will be required to be able to *grip*.

Think about all of the steps required to complete the activity. Look back at your analysis of the body functions required for the activity; this can direct you toward identifying the performance skills needed. For example, decorating a cake requires a high level of fine and gross motor coordination, eye-hand coordination, and strength in the hands; thus the motor skills are in high demand. However, this activity requires little to no social interaction skills, as there are typically no steps in decorating a cake that require interaction with others.

The objects used, the environment, and the social demands all contribute to the extent to which specific performance skills are required. It is for this reason that determining the performance skills is not done earlier in the activity analysis process. The identification of these aspects of the activity demands first provides a link to understanding the performance skill required in each area. The size, shape, and sensory qualities of the objects that are used determine the level of skill. For example, in washing the hands using bar soap, there is a high demand for the motor skills of *manipulates* and *grips* to assure that the bar of soap stays in the hands and does not slip out onto the floor. If during the activity analysis it is determined that liquid soap in a bottle, with a pump dispenser, would be used, there would less of a demand for *manipulates* and more for *aligns, positions,* and *moves*. As you can see, a change in an object greatly changes the demand for client skill.

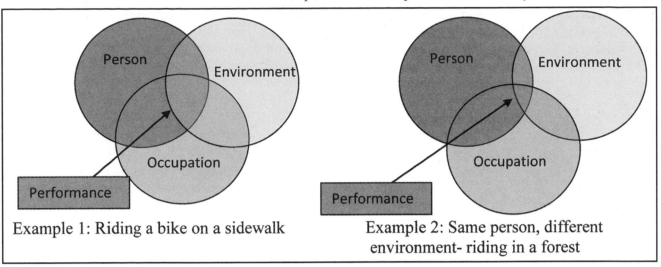

Figure 8-1. The PEO model: influence of the person, environment, and occupation on performance.

As you are determining the performance skills required of the activity you are analyzing, think also about the environment in which the activity takes place. The surface and space may influence the required skill. For example, a low level of motor and process skill is needed to go down a beginner ski slope versus the skill level needed for an expert slope.

The social demands of the activity may also have an impact on the skill level required. If we are analyzing the activity of playing a board game, the social demands are important to understand before determining the performance skills. How many other players are going to be playing? Are there specific rules for this game? Are there specific unspoken rules within the group of people playing the game? What are the expectations of performance from the players? What level of interaction between the players is expected? The answers to these questions will influence the extent to which not only the *social interaction skills* are required but also the *process* and *motor skills*. A game in which each player is expected to make his or her move within a 30-second time frame will require a higher level of process skills, such as *paces, attends, chooses, initiates, continues, terminates, searches/ locates, notices/responds*, and others, depending on the actual game.

Ecological models and theories—such as the Ecology of Human Performance model, the Person-Environment-Occupational Performance model, and the Person-Environment-Occupation (PEO) model—support the principles used to determine the performance skills demanded of an activity. These models contend that the ability to perform in an occupation is influenced not only by the aspects of the person (body functions, beliefs, values), but also by the aspects of the occupation (the objects and properties, social demands, sequence, and timing) and the environment (the space demands and physical context). Using this frame to understand performance, the skill level needed to perform an activity is measured not only by the body functions utilized, but also by the activity and the environment in which the activity is performed. As the environment changes, the skill level may have to increase or decrease. For example, the skill level needed to ride a bike increases when the surface and environment become more complex, as when one is riding on a dirt path as opposed to a city street.

In the PEO model (Figure 8-1), the area in the center of the diagram where all three circles overlap indicates the performance of the occupation being engaged in. As one of the areas moves or changes— as in the example of biking, where the environment changes—the demand for skill level increases and that for performance decreases. This demonstrates the view that performance is influenced not only by skill and body functions, but also by the activity itself and the contexts in which it is performed.

MOTOR SKILLS

Motor skills are "observed as the person interacts with and moves task objects and self around the task environment (Boyt Schell, Gillen, & Scaffa, 2014, p. 1237)" (AOTA, 2014, p. S25). These are the movement-related skills that are used to move and interact with the environment and objects in it.

TABLE 8-1
SPECIFIC MOTOR SKILLS RELATED TO BODY POSITION

Aligns	Moves
Stabilizes	Lifts
Positions	Walks
Reaches	Transports
Bends	Calibrates
Grips	Flows
Manipulates	Endures
Coordinates	Paces

As mentioned earlier, the objects and their properties influence not only the skills required, but also the extent to which they are challenged during performance of the activity. If the objects being used become more difficult to maneuver (e.g., using small buttons versus big buttons), then the skills of manipulates and coordinates will be more needed. If the physical environment provides greater challenges, then the requirements for greater control over motor-related skills will increase. The social expectations and demands may also influence the skill level required of an activity. For example, if you were writing a note to yourself, the motor/praxis skill needed would be low because there is no social expectation for legibility. However, if you were writing an address on an envelope that will be going into the mail, a moderate level of motor/praxis skill would be required as the address must be read by the workers in the post office.

Motor skills require the utilization of several body functions, many of which work in conjunction with each other to produce purposeful movement (Table 8-1). Of course, simply having a body function does not imply skill level or ability (AOTA, 2014). Motor skills are units of action that are observable and utilize a variety of body functions.

Aligns

The skill of aligns is defined as when the participant "interacts with task objects without evidence of persistent propping or persistent leaning" (AOTA, 2014, p. S25). We align our bodies into position when we interact with objects or move so that we can efficiently

and appropriately interact with the objects required of the activity. For example, in making scrambled eggs, you must align your body and keep it upright when the pan is lifted up, the eggs are broken using both hands, and the eggs are stirred in the pan. Aligning the body requires that the person not prop themselves up or lean. While sitting in class, a student is required to demonstrate a level of ability to align his or her body in the chair. However, if you are at home right now, sitting reading this book on a couch, there may little demand for you to align your body.

Stabilizes

Stabilization of the body occurs when a person moves through the environment and interacts with objects, all without propping or a loss of balance (AOTA, 2014). We are challenged to stabilize our bodies against gravity and the environment when we are moving. When you walk through a store and reach for a box of cereal off the shelf, you are stabilizing your body to keep from falling.

Positions

People position themselves when they must establish an "effective distance from task objects and without evidence of awkward body positioning" (AOTA, 2014, p. S25). The position of our body in relation to the objects we are working with and the environment we are engaging with affects the performance of the activity. For example, while making scrambled eggs, you need to crack open the eggshells. In order for this to occur, you position your body in front of the bowl or pan into which you will place the eggs. Imagine if you were to crack the eggshells and then have to reach far away from your body in order to place the eggs in a bowl. The result would probably be messy.

Making Sense of Aligns, Stabilizes, and Positions

To clarify the difference between the three performance skills related to body position, let us take a look at the activity of golf. In attempting to hit the ball from a tee, the participant must first position himself in front of the ball so that he can reach the ball with his club when he swings. Once in position, he must align

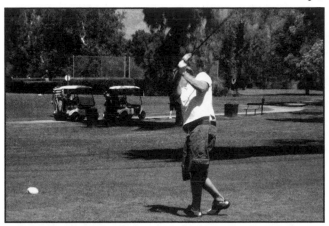

Figure 8-2. When a golfer takes a swing at the ball, he aligns, stabilizes, and positions his body.

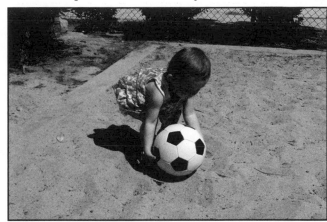

Figure 8-3. June bends over to pick up a ball.

his body so that he can use the club to effectively make contact with the ball. He might align his shoulders in a certain way and align his feet to align with his hips and shoulders. As he swings the club, he stabilizes his body keep from losing his balance and falling over as he twists and turns (Figure 8-2).

MOTOR SKILLS RELATED TO OBTAINING AND HOLDING OBJECTS

Reaches

During everyday activities, the objects we utilize and engage with are often positioned away from the body and require us to extend our arms in order to interact with them. This may also require bending the trunk in order to effectively reach an item or object (AOTA, 2014). Think about how much you reach every day. When you woke up, you may have reached over to turn off your alarm clock, reached to open the shower curtain or door, reached into the shower to turn on the water, reached to pick up soap and shampoo, and so on.

Bends

In order to reach or grasp an object, a person may be required to flex or rotate the trunk. This requires her to bend to grasp or place objects that are out of reach (AOTA, 2014). Bending is also required in interacting

with objects such as chairs. You must bend your trunk in order to sit or get up. Bending to reach or engage with an object can also occur through trunk rotation, as when passing papers to a person sitting behind you in a classroom (Figure 8-3).

Grips

The skill of gripping is the effective use of the fingers, teeth, toes, or other body parts to pinch or hold onto objects, not allowing them to slip (AOTA, 2014). A gymnast might grip a parallel bar with her legs; a golfer would grip the golf club with his hands. In the activity of making scrambled eggs, the ability to grip is required for holding the handle of the pan, holding the eggs, and gripping the handle of the spatula when stirring the eggs (Figure 8-4).

Manipulates

The skill of manipulates is defined as "uses dexterous finger movements, without evidence of fumbling, when manipulating task objects" (AOTA, 2014, p. S25). The ability to manipulate is greatly influenced by the body function of control of voluntary movement, specifically fine motor control. Manipulating objects using the fingers is required for activities such as typing, using a cell phone, and buttoning buttons. In making scrambled eggs, the skill of manipulating is utilized when handling the eggs and cracking them in half, pulling the shells carefully apart (Figure 8-5).

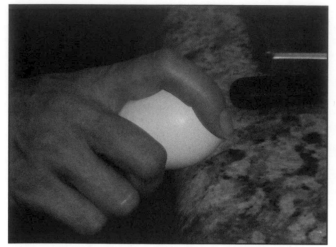

Figure 8-4. Gripping an egg while making scrambled eggs.

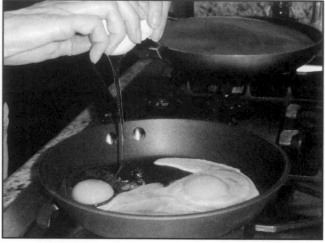

Figure 8-5. Manipulating the two parts of an eggshell to open it.

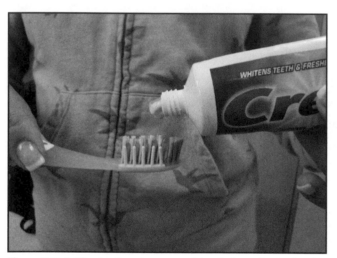

Figure 8-6. Putting toothpaste on a toothbrush through coordination of both hands.

Coordinates

The use of two or more body parts together to utilize an object requires the skill of coordinates. Coordination requires the synchronization of body parts to work together to manipulate or steady objects being used during an activity without fumbling or dropping them (AOTA, 2014). For example, in brushing a dog, one hand is used to hold the dog still while the other is used to hold the brush and move it over the dog's fur. When we prepare to brush our teeth, one hand holds the toothbrush while the other holds the toothpaste and applies it to the bristles of the brush (Figure 8-6). Without the coordination of both hands, you might end up with toothpaste everywhere except on the toothbrush.

MOTOR SKILLS RELATED TO MOVING SELF AND OBJECTS

Moves

We move objects by either pushing or pulling them along a surface (AOTA, 2014) (Figure 8-7). For example, we move the pedals of a bike by pushing them along their axis. We pull our chairs in underneath us when sitting at a table by scooting them along the floor. A client might move a front-wheeled walker by pushing it along the floor. Pushing the wheels of a wheelchair allows a person to move it forward, backward, or to the side.

Lifts

To lift means to raise or elevate objects required of the activity "without evidence of increased effort" (AOTA, 2014, p. S23). We lift objects in order to utilize them or to organize our environment and make space within it. For example, you might lift weeds out of a garden, lift your toothbrush up to your mouth, or lift a golf club out of a golf bag. Another way of thinking of the skill of lifting is to think of the action of picking up something. For example, a mother might pick her child's toys up from the floor to keep from tripping over them.

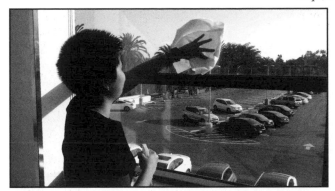

Figure 8-7. In cleaning windows, the cloth is moved across the glass.

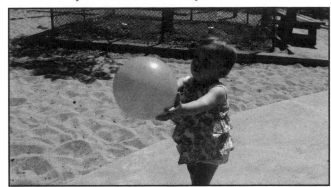

Figure 8-8. June carrying or transporting a ball from one place to another.

Walks

OT professionals look at walking from the perspective of how it is used in the context of daily occupations. Skilled walking, while engaging in an occupation, includes ambulating on a surface without shuffling the feet, using an assistive device (such as a walker or cane), or becoming unstable (AOTA, 2014). Many occupations require that a person ambulate from one position to another, such as cooking and walking from one area of a kitchen to another to obtain and use items. There are many activities where this skill is required, but the skill level required varies according to the activity and how much smooth unassisted walking is required. Activities that require someone to have a high level of walking skill, where he or she must move smoothly and without loss of balance, are activities such as competitive sports activities or modeling.

Transports

Transporting objects entails carrying objects needed for an activity from one place to another while moving by walking or using a wheelchair (AOTA, 2014). This requires the use of our upper extremities to carry objects while maneuvering around in the environment or from one environment to another (Figure 8-8). For example, during the activity of feeding a dog, the participant must carry the food dish to an area from a place in which the meal is prepared to a place in which the dog will eat. This may be a few feet away or in a completely different environment (from inside to outside the home). Another example of when the skill of transports is required is while doing laundry. The dirty laundry must be carried and transported from one area of the home to where the washing machine is located.

Calibrates

To calibrate movement means to use appropriate force when interacting with an object. It also includes calibrating the appropriate speed or the extent of the movement when using or coming in contact with an object (AOTA, 2014). For example, when you hold hands with someone, you must calibrate the force with which we grasp the other person's hand as well as how hard you hold it. To use the example of golf again, the participant must calibrate the speed of acceleration and deceleration of the movement of the golf club.

Flows

The action of flow is the use of "smooth and fluid arm and wrist movements when interacting with task objects" (AOTA, 2014, p. S25). When we are utilizing objects during participation in an activity, the ability to move smoothly is often essential to completion of the activity or for safety. For example, when using a curling iron to curl hair, the person using the curling iron must pick it up smoothly and move it toward the hair smoothly. He or she must use careful and fluid movements of the arm and wrist in order to produce the desired results and also to assure that the skin or hair is not burned. When we are engaging in activities, we flow from one movement to another, shifting direction and stopping movement smoothly. In brushing your teeth, you use smooth, fluid movements to bring the brush to your mouth and then control the wrist and arm movements as you move it from one part of your mouth to the other. So, in analyzing an

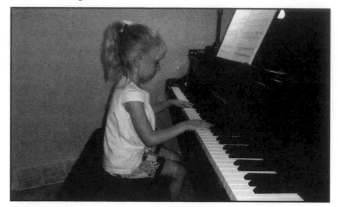

Figure 8-9. Playing the piano requires pacing of movements.

activity, think about the movements that require the person to move smoothly and fluidly from one direction to another or to control direction in the middle of movement. This skill is especially important when accuracy of smooth movements influences success in the occupation or activity. Also consider the safety considerations of the activity and if the participant's ability to flow impacts safety. What objects are utilized or interacted with during the activity? Does the participant pick up and move these objects? If the movements are not smooth and fluid, are there safety risks? Would the participant be successful in the activity if he or she were not able to move smoothly or fluidly while moving the object(s) or when moving from one direction to the next? These are all questions to ask in determining the extent to which the performance skill of flow is required for an activity.

Motor Skills Related to Sustaining Performance

Endures

To endure requires the participant to persist through a task without "obvious evidence of physical fatigue, pausing to rest, or stopping to catch one's breath" (AOTA, 2014, p. S25). The extent to which a client must physically endure aspects of an activity depends on the length of the activity and the extent to which continuous physical activity is required for each step. An activity may require a person to physically engage for several minutes and then require the person to stop, which provides an opportunity for rest of the body. For other activities, continuous movement or physical activity may be required for a prolonged period of time, challenging the person's ability to endure. For example, washing hair in the shower requires the person to endure about 5 to 10 minutes of standing in the shower and moving the upper extremities to apply soap, scrub, and then rinse. The demand for endurance is minimal but nonetheless essential to the process. In contrast, the endurance needed for preparing a four-course meal is much greater, as the person is required to be standing and moving for a much longer period of time, with few opportunities for rest. In determining the extent to which the performance skill of endures is required of an activity, look at the steps and the length of time the person is required to move. Is the participant required to be moving continuously without pausing to rest or catching her breath? Are there rest breaks inherent in the activity, where the person stops physical activity for more process or cognitively oriented tasks?

Paces

In engaging in activities that require motor skills, pacing involves the ability to maintain a consistent tempo or rate of movement during the task (AOTA, 2014) (Figure 8-9). This ability to pace is important when motor movements must occur at a certain rate, such as a certain number of repetitions within a certain amount of time, or at a certain tempo, with movements occurring at certain speeds. A perfect example of this is with dancing. Movements occur at a certain rate and tempo as the dancers pace their movements according to the music. We pace ourselves during other daily activities such as driving; we turn the steering wheel at a certain pace when turning a corner to assure we turn safely and accurately. We walk into a building at a certain pace or rate in order to get to school or work on time. We might speed up or slow down our movements based on need. If making scrambled eggs, the participant must maintain a certain rate of movement when whipping the eggs in a bowl in order to effectively mix the eggs. If we must get a task done in a certain amount of time, such as getting ready to go to school or work in the morning, we must pace our movements in order to complete each task at a certain rate. If we did not pace our movements, we might never get anywhere on time or complete activities effectively.

Process Skills

Process skills are those observable actions in which the participant "(1) selects, interacts with, and uses task tools and materials; (2) carries out individual actions and steps; and (3) modifies performance when problems are encountered" (Boyt Schell et al., 2014a, p. 1239; AOTA, 2014, S25). These are the skills that require mental functions, both specific and global. It is within process skills that understanding and perceiving the sensory information we receive from our surroundings is utilized. Process skills allow us to plan and manage our way through the steps of an activity and respond to changes in the environment as they occur. They allow us to select the appropriate objects and environment for the activity and the appropriate time to conduct the activity. Process skills also allow us to identify problems and solutions to the problems and to be creative and multitask. Twenty process skills are identified in the *Framework* (Table 8-2).

Paces

If this term looks familiar, it is because it was also described as a motor skill. Thus, when identifying paces as a performance skill, it is important to designate if it is the process skill of paces or the motor skill of paces. The process skill of pacing is also maintaining a consistent rate or tempo throughout a task, but in this case it is the mental process of pacing the task (AOTA, 2014). The participant must choose the tempo and pace of the actions and steps to assure that the activity or occupation is completed in the time required, or at a tempo which is demanded for successful completion of the task. For example, to take an exam for a class, the participants must pace themselves, answering questions at a certain rate in order to complete the exam on time. We often pace ourselves without conscious thought, as when eating. In determining the extent to which the process skill of pacing is required, think about the time demands of certain steps. Do tasks need to be done within a certain time frame? Do tasks need to be completed at a certain tempo, such as one per minute?

TABLE 8-2 PROCESS SKILLS	
Paces	Terminates
Attends	Searches/locates
Heeds	Gathers
Chooses	Organizes
Uses	Restores
Handles	Navigates
Inquires	Notices/responds
Initiates	Adjusts
Continues	Accommodates
Sequences	Benefits

Attends

To attend requires the participant to pay direct attention to what he is doing, without looking away or interrupting continuous engagement (AOTA, 2014). The level of attention required for activities varies and is greatly influenced by safety and time expectations. For example, completing an examination within a certain time frame requires a high level of the skill to attend to the task. At the other end of the continuum of demand for attention lie activities such as eating a snack, listening to music, or surfing the Internet. Even activities such as watching television require some level of attention in order to understand and follow what is occurring in what is being watched. If the participant is surfing television shows and changing channels frequently, this requires very little attention as sustained or continuous engagement is not required. In determining the extent to which the ability to attend is required, think about how long the participant must direct his attention to the task without looking away or interrupting their engagement with the task.

Heeds

To heed is to carry out and complete a task that was agreed upon or specified by another person (AOTA,

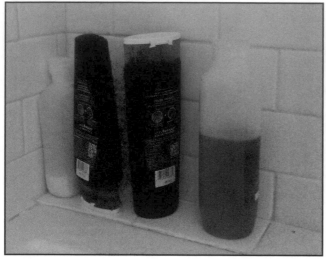

Figure 8-10. In washing one's hair, one must choose the proper amount of shampoo.

2014). This skill requires that the participant complete an activity or task as it was designed or specified to be completed. This means that they must continue on through the steps until successful completion, as defined by the participant prior to initiation of the task or by another person. For example, an instructor may ask a student to write a 10-page paper on activity analysis (what a fun topic!). To heed would mean that the student must continue to write the paper until it is completed, heeding all directions given (attending to the directions) and providing 10 pages of written material. This skill is important when activities need to be completed in a specific way or completion is defined by another person.

PROCESS SKILLS RELATED TO APPLYING KNOWLEDGE

Chooses

When a person chooses during an activity, he or she is selecting the tools, choosing the appropriate type and number of tools, and selecting the appropriate type of materials needed for the activity. This also includes selecting the tools and materials that another person directed them to use or was specified that they would use (AOTA, 2014). This requires attending to what is known about the activity and what objects (and their properties) are needed in order to complete the activity. For example, when shampooing your hair

in the shower, you would need to choose the shampoo and choose the appropriate amount of shampoo in order to successfully wash your hair (Figure 8-10). In determining whether this skill is required for an activity, think about the objects that are utilized during the activity. Does the participant need to choose to use those objects? Are there a variety of objects in the environment to choose from? Does the participant need to determine the particular type of object to be used? Does he or she need to determine the amount or number of objects or materials being used or to choose the objects or materials as directed?

Uses

The skill of using occurs when the participant utilizes tools and materials appropriately and as intended. This also means that objects are used safely and in a hygienic fashion (AOTA, 2014). For example, a person would use a toothbrush to brush his teeth, not his hair. This skill is demanded when there are objects utilized during the activity that would pose safety hazards if not used properly, or they may pose hygiene issues, or the activity may be done incorrectly or not completed. How a client uses objects and materials influences successful engagement in occupations. An activity requires the skill of uses when there are objects or materials involved in the activity that the participant must actively utilize. The demand for this skill increases if the objects must be used in a specific way or if there are safety or hygiene dangers if the objects are not used appropriately.

Handles

The process skill of handling objects requires the person to support or stabilize tools and materials "in an appropriate manner, protecting them from being damaged, slipping, moving, and falling" (AOTA, 2014, p. S25). For many activities, successful participation relies on the participant's ability to handle the objects being used. For example, in the activity of making scrambled eggs, the person must understand how to handle the eggs in order to keep them from breaking prematurely. Because this is a process skill and not a motor skill, it is important to note that this is the mental skill of understanding how to handle objects and then executing the activity based on that understanding. A person demonstrating this skill would handle a variety of objects differently, based on what he or she knew of the activity and the objects and their properties. We handle and protect objects on a daily basis. In picking up grocery bags, you might grasp the bags from the bottom to keep them from ripping or slipping from your grasp and falling to the floor. Instead of throwing the grocery bags into the kitchen, we handle the bags more carefully and set them onto a counter or table.

Inquires

A person uses the skill of inquires when he or she seeks out and requests needed verbal or written information and "does not ask for information when he or she was fully oriented to the task and environment and had immediate prior awareness" (AOTA, 2014, S25). This includes seeking out information by asking someone questions or reading written information when needed. A person inquires when appropriate, when he or she is not familiar with the activity or task, or has not been fully oriented to the activity or environment (the activity or environment are new to the person). Any new activity may require the participant to inquire for more information. For example, when given an assignment to complete, a student might inquire for further information from the written directions or ask questions of the instructor. In this era of information via technology, many inquiries can be made online. We might be engaging in a new occupation, such as gardening, and we search online for what plants are best to plant in our specific geographical location. Activities that require the acquisition of new information or where the activity is new to the participant will require this process skill. Activities that are familiar but are being performed in a new environment or with unfamiliar objects may require the participant to make inquiries.

PROCESS SKILLS RELATED TO TEMPORAL ORGANIZATION

Initiates

To initiate requires that the participant start each step or action required of the activity without hesitation (AOTA, 2014). This means that they start or begin each step of the activity smoothly and without

pausing. When we begin an activity, we initiate the first step with an action, but then we must continue to initiate as we move from one step to another. For example, during the activity of brushing her teeth, the participant must initiate picking up the toothbrush in one hand. She must then initiate picking up the toothpaste, then initiate taking the cap off of the toothpaste, and so on. Each step of an activity requires the participant to initiate action.

Continues

The skill of continues is seen when the participant must perform actions without interruption. Once an activity is initiated, the participant continues without pauses or delays until the action is completed (AOTA, 2014). The action or skill of continuing allows for completion of an activity or for greater effectiveness. For example, in washing your hair in the shower, you must continue to rinse out the shampoo until your hair is free of residual suds, otherwise the task is not completed correctly. Activities that require the skill of continues are those involving steps that the participant must perform or a continuous action for a specific amount of time without interruption.

Sequences

To sequence is to perform the steps of a task in a logical and effective order. The demonstration of this skill requires that there is no randomness in the ordering of steps or inappropriate repetition of actions or steps (AOTA, 2014). The sequencing of an activity is a mental processing skill that entails determining the appropriate progression of an activity prior to or during engagement in the activity, shaping the course of the activity by choosing which action takes place after another. Most activities require some level of sequencing. Activities that involve multiple steps in a specific order require a higher level of this skill.

Terminates

Concluding an activity at the appropriate time and without persistence beyond what is safe or suitable for the activity requires the skill of being able to terminate. This also includes stopping specific steps or actions within a task (AOTA, 2014). Without the skill of termination, we might continue activities too long, not stopping until damage occurs or we can no longer continue. This skill is essential to the efficient and accurate completion of activities and crucial to ensuring safety. For example, a person who is brushing her teeth must know when to terminate the brushing actions, otherwise damage to the gums, the insides of the cheeks, and the teeth can occur. Termination is a skill required for most activities, but it is required at a much higher level for those activities in which safety would be compromised if the participant did not stop or terminate the action at the appropriate time. It is also highly required for those activities that comprise multiple steps and rely on the conclusion of one step in order to move forward with the next.

PROCESS SKILLS RELATED TO ORGANIZING SPACE AND OBJECTS

Searches/Locates

To search and locate requires the participant to scan the environment, either visually or tactilely, to locate objects and materials. Searching must occur in a logical manner, looking within and outside of the immediate environment (AOTA, 2014). An example of this might be when you try to find your keys. You might look around your home environment and feel around in your bags for the keys. If they were not found, you might venture out and search other places where they might be, such as outside the door, in the door, in a car, or at a friend's house. On an everyday level, you search and locate items during most of your daily self-care activities. Think of your morning routine and how often you must scan the environment and locate the objects with which you interact. When you brushed your teeth, you looked (and perhaps felt) around for your toothbrush and the toothpaste. While the searching is probably not too difficult if you keep it in the same place every day, it still requires you to scan your environment to locate the needed objects. Activities that involve the use of objects will require the skill of searches and locates. The greater the number of objects and the complexity of their location, the more the skill will be required.

Gathers

Collecting the needed tools and materials into the space being used for the activity being engaged in requires the ability to gather. Gathering encompasses not only assembling all of the needed tools and materials together, but also cleaning up materials that have spilled or fallen and replacing objects that have been misplaced (AOTA, 2014). For example, the skill of gathers is used during the activity of cooking. In order to begin the activity of making scrambled eggs, the participant must gather the eggs, pan, spatula, and oil and bring them to the stove (the work space). This skill is required of activities in which objects or materials must be collected and brought to a specific work area or environment. Examples of activities that require the skill of gathering are gardening, skiing, and shopping.

Organizes

When a person organizes, she is demonstrating the ability to logically arrange or position the objects used during an activity in a way that facilitates engagement and is not too crowded yet not too spread out. The organization of the objects must occur in the space or spaces in which the activity takes place (AOTA, 2014). Let's use the activity of writing a paper as an example. If a student is writing a paper on activity analysis, she might organize her work space by placing books, papers, reading glasses (if needed), a cup of coffee or tea, pens, pencils, and scratch paper around her within reach, so that they could easily be utilized while she was typing on the computer. The extent to which an activity requires the participant to organize depends on the extent to which objects are utilized and how efficiently the participant can reach for them. If an activity needs to be done quickly and efficiently, the demand for the ability to organize increases. However, the number or existence of objects does not necessarily determine the need to organize. For some activities, there is little need to organize the objects during the activity. For example, when making a cup of tea, there is very little demand for the participant to organize the objects when engaging in the activity. The requirement for organization may also lie in the social demands of the activity, where the expectations of others guide how much the participant must organize. An unorganized desk might be acceptable in some work environments, while in others, a desk must be organized in a way that facilitates easy and efficient access to needed materials (without digging through piles of papers).

Restores

Putting away the objects, tools, and materials used during an activity is the skill of being able to restore. This encompasses putting away objects in their appropriate places and restoring the area where the activity took place to its original state (AOTA, 2014). For example, when you are washing your hair in the shower, you put the shampoo back where it was found, turn off the shower, and close the shower door or curtain so that the space is restored to a condition in which it is ready to be used again. We return objects back to their respective places throughout our day and to varying levels. When we write down a message, we might retrieve a pen and paper, write it down, and then return the pen and paper back to where they came from. A greater level of restoring occurs when it is not just small objects that must be returned to a proper place but rather an environment that must be brought back to a certain state. An example would be the actions required after hosting a party. We must place all trash in trash bins, move furniture, remove dirt or liquid from the floor or table tops, and return serving plates or silverware to their respective places, as well as countless other random things that you might find after hosting a party (it depends on how wild this party was). The extent to which the skill of restoring is required is linked to the number of objects utilized during the activity, the extent to which they are displaced from their original storing area, and the social demands related to restoring the environment to a specific state.

Navigates

When people navigate, they are moving through the environment in which the activity takes place and interacting with objects, moving their arms, bodies, or wheelchair without bumping into objects or people (AOTA, 2014). Navigating is the process skill of determining how to move within a space without colliding or interacting with others or objects. When we move around in our environment, moving our arms, legs, and bodies, we are continuously making decisions about how to move and how to assure our safety. Think of when you got up out of bed this morning. You sat up and probably walked to the bathroom (just a guess; it is usually a person's first stop in the morning). In order to successfully get to the bathroom, you had to navigate around the bed and through the environment to make sure that you did not bump into anything, hurting yourself or something in the environment (such as stepping on a cat). When determining the extent to which the skill of navigating is required for an activity, think about how much the person has to move throughout the activity. Does he need to move around objects or move his entire body through space? Does he need to avoid objects as he moves his arms or legs? An example of this is in putting dishes away in a cupboard—the person must move her arms through space, navigating her arm and hand around the doors and shelves of the cupboard.

PROCESS SKILLS RELATED TO ADAPTING PERFORMANCE

Notices/Responds

The ability to notice or respond requires the participant to react appropriately to cues provided by the task at hand or the spatial arrangement or alignment of objects being used in the activity. All of these cues are visual, auditory, tactile, or temperature cues provided by the environment or objects, not a person (they do not include verbal cues) (AOTA, 2014). For example, in making scrambled eggs, the participant notices the eggs hardening in the pan and stirs them. He might feel the heat of the pan near his hand and move away to avoid being burned. He might notice a drawer open in the kitchen and close it. We utilize our ability to notice and respond in many activities throughout the day. It allows for safe and effective performance of activities. Without noticing and responding to moving objects, unsafe environments, or objects that are safety concerns, we put ourselves at risk for injury or possibly even death. Think of when you are driving or riding a bike. You must notice and respond to cars or other vehicles in your path, otherwise you might be hit or might hit someone else. The ability to notice and respond is a skill that is required for many activities in which we must use our sensory abilities to obtain and process information and respond to that information.

Activities that require the participant to take action based on things occurring in the environment or to respond to objects being utilized during the activity (such as the position of objects in relation to the participant or other objects) require the skill of being able to notice/respond.

Adjusts

During engagement in an activity, the skill of being able to adjust is often essential to successful participation. Adjusting is the action of moving to a different work area, using different tools or materials, or adjusting objects in the environment to overcome challenges or problems faced during engagement in the activity (AOTA, 2014). As a process skill, this is the volitional choice a participant makes to change environments or the objects when faced with difficulties. For example, if a student was trying to study at school and the room in which she was studying was too noisy, she would adjust by moving to another room to study (taking all of her books and study materials with her). Adjusting implies not only moving environments, but also adjusting the objects we are using. For example, in washing your hair in the shower, you might adjust the water temperature in order to supply water that will be neither too hot nor too cold. Activities that require the skill of being able to adjust are those in which the environment or objects and materials can change. Does the participant have the freedom to choose and change environments if problems arise? Can adjustments be made to the objects or materials being used? Are there potential challenges or problems that can occur during the activity that will require the participant to adjust to those challenges?

Accommodates

During engagement in activities, we often must accommodate, or change our actions, in order to prevent errors or ineffective performance (AOTA, 2014). To accommodate means to make room for, or to adapt (*Mosby's Dictionary of Medicine*, 2006). Activities that require us to accommodate are those that present themselves with varying conditions, or the potential for changing conditions during the activity. In order to assure success, we must be able to adjust and accommodate to those changes or challenges. For example, if during the activity of grocery shopping you find that your shopping cart has a defective wheel and

does not steer straight, you accommodate by pushing the cart differently in order to avoid knocking over everything in the store with the cart. We adjust our actions to avoid errors every day, without conscious effort. When you find that the road you usually take to work or school is closed for construction, you must accommodate and change your path. If a friend calls while you are studying and desperately needs to talk, you accommodate by adjusting your schedule to make the needed time.

Benefits

When an error or problem occurs, we benefit from those events by preventing those problems from occurring again or allowing them to continue (AOTA, 2014). Our ability to process why problems occur and how to avoid them in the future is a skill that ensures future success in activities which have the potential for challenges. For example, if during the activity of making scrambled eggs the participant breaks the egg too forcefully and the egg crumbles, he or she will benefit from that experience by making sure that the egg is broken more gently the next time. The skill of benefits is utilized during activities where the participant learns from actions and uses those experiences to prevent failure or ineffective task performance.

SOCIAL INTERACTION SKILLS

According to the *Framework*, social interactions are "observed during the ongoing stream of a social exchange" (AOTA, 2014, p. S26). The social interaction skills listed in the *Framework* are based on the skills included in the Evaluation of Social Interaction assessment by Fisher and Griswold (2008). In this assessment tool, the authors present seven categories of social interaction skills, all of which can either support or hinder successful engagement in occupations (Simmons, Griswold, & Brett, 2010). Interacting socially and communicating our needs and thoughts effectively is a skill that is gained over time. On a daily basis, we are interacting with others either directly or indirectly, as in writing a paper or sending a text message.

The behaviors we exhibit in interacting with others are part of our social interaction skills. How we act and behave when around others is part of what we are

TABLE 8-3
SOCIAL INTERACTION SKILLS

Approaches/starts	Regulates	Times duration
Concludes/disengages	Questions	Takes turns
Produces speech	Replies	Matches language
Gesticulates	Discloses	Clarifies
Speaks fluently	Expresses emotion	Acknowledges and encourages
Turns toward	Disagrees	Empathizes
Looks	Thanks	Heeds
Places self	Transitions	Accommodates
Touches	Times response	Benefits

communicating to others about ourselves. Maintaining the appropriate physical space between the listener and speaker is a social skill. Initiating appropriate conversation, taking turns, and responding appropriately to a speaker are also social skills. Think of someone with whom your interaction felt awkward or you felt that he or she had poor social skills. What behaviors did this person demonstrate that made you feel uncomfortable? Was his or her choice of topic inappropriate? Did he or she make rude bodily noises during conversation? Did this person use foul language? Perhaps he or she looked away and was distracted by the environment while you talked. All of these are examples of how the lack of social interaction skills can detract from the effectiveness of communication.

The social interaction skills required of an activity are very much reliant on the social demands for that particular activity. For example, the social demands, and thus the social skills, needed for bowling with friends would be very different from those needed for bowling in a tournament. Thus the language, use of physical space, touching, body language, turn taking, and personal acknowledgments used during conversations can vary widely according to the setting and social demands. It is not uncommon for a person to use one set of social interaction skills in one setting and quite a different set while in another. Do you communicate the same way while at school as you do at home with friends or family?

Social interaction skills go beyond the face-to-face and in-person interactions. Social interaction skills are also utilized when on the telephone and in conducting online communications. The use of certain abbreviations (e.g., LOL for "laugh out loud") has become an acceptable way of communicating in text messaging, instant messaging, or e-mail. Thus it is important to remember that communication and social skills are utilized in a variety of settings, including virtual environments (Table 8-3).

SOCIAL INTERACTION SKILLS RELATED TO INITIATING AND TERMINATING SOCIAL INTERACTION

Approaches/Starts

Approaching or starting involves initiating an interaction with another person in a socially appropriate manner (AOTA, 2014). The social demands of the specific activity will define what is socially appropriate and acceptable in regard to initiating a conversation or interaction. Approaching another person and starting an interaction can occur in many activities and in a variety of contexts. It can occur not only face-to-face, but also in the virtual context. In some web-based contexts, it is appropriate to initiate a conversation with a stranger, while in others it is not.

Concludes/Disengages

Concluding and disengaging a conversation or interaction is a skill that entails effectively ending a conversation or social interaction. This requires that the participant conclude the discussion by bringing

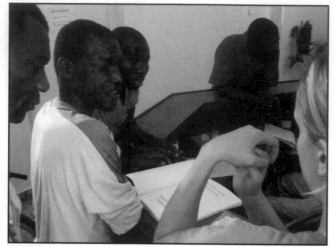

Figure 8-11. An occupational therapy student teaches Haitians medical information using body language.

closure to the topic and saying goodbye to the person or people involved (AOTA, 2014). This skill is required for verbal and written communication or interactions.

SOCIAL INTERACTION SKILLS RELATED TO PRODUCING SOCIAL INTERACTION

Produces Speech

Producing speech can occur through spoken word, sign language, or the use of a computer-generated device. Producing speech requires that what is being generated during the interaction is audible and articulated clearly (AOTA, 2014). The exception to this is in the case of the use of sign language, in which the production of the signs must be done clearly.

Gesticulates

When we communicate or interact with others, we use not only our words, but also the movement of our bodies to demonstrate our thoughts and needs. This is the ability to gesticulate: to use gestures in a socially appropriate way to communicate (AOTA, 2014). How you move your arms, head, and trunk during conversation provides an extra element to your interactions.

Try having a conversation with someone with your hands behind your back and without moving your head. You will find how essential this skill is to effective interactions. This skill is especially important for activities in which the participant is trying to explain something, give directions, or convey an important message (Figure 8-11).

Speaks Fluently

Speaking fluently is a skill in which the speaker speaks fluidly, in an articulate and continuous manner, and at an even pace. Speaking fluently also includes speaking without inappropriate pauses or lulls throughout (AOTA, 2014). There are many activities in which speaking fluently is required, but not at a high level, as when talking with an old friend or family member. However, in delivering a speech or presentation, the ability to speak fluently at a high level is required.

SOCIAL INTERACTION SKILLS RELATED TO PHYSICALLY SUPPORTING SOCIAL INTERACTION

Turns Toward

Much of what we convey when we interact with others occurs through our body language and how we position ourselves in relation to the other person or group of people. When a person turns toward, she is actively turning her body and face to position herself toward the other person who is speaking (AOTA, 2014). Socially, this is a sign that the person is engaged in the interaction and actively participating. Imagine if you were to engage in a conversation with someone in front of you and instead of turning around and facing you, the individual spoke to you while facing forward. This would seem very strange, right? In order to engage in an interaction or conversation, we physically position ourselves so that we can see the other person and they can see us. This skill is required for any face-to-face interaction in which the people involved have the freedom to move their bodies and heads.

Looks

Another manner in which we communicate and interact using body language is by looking at or making eye contact with a social partner (AOTA, 2014). Making eye contact occurs when the participant looks at the eyes of the social partner. This can occur throughout the interaction but does not need to occur continuously. The amount of eye contact required of a participant during an activity or interaction depends on the social demands of the activity. For example, during a job interview, the participant should look at the interviewer and provide good eye contact.

Places Self

Have you ever had a conversation with someone who positioned himself too close to you during the interaction? Placing the self in an appropriate position and at a proper distance is an important aspect of communication and interaction. This is the skill of placing yourself at a socially acceptable distance and position from the other person or people who are part of the interaction (AOTA, 2014). The extent to which this skill is required is very much reliant on the social demands of the activity and what is socially acceptable to those engaging in the interaction.

Touches

The use of touch during conversations can either support or hinder the success of an interaction. Participants must be able to accept the touch of others as well as touch or make bodily contact with others in a socially acceptable manner (AOTA, 2014). Just as with many of the other social interaction skills in this section, what is socially acceptable during interactions is very dependent on the social demands of the activity and the culture of the participants (Figure 8-12).

Regulates

During a social interaction, regulating is preventing repetitive, impulsive, or irrelevant behaviors that are not part of the message being conveyed (AOTA, 2014). Regulating behavior during social interaction is important in interacting with others who have expectations of certain behaviors or the interaction

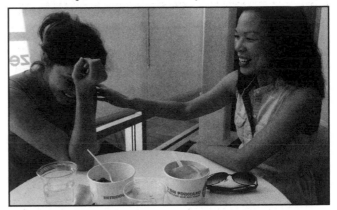

Figure 8-12. We often use touch to communicate unspoken feelings.

is occurring in a public place. For example, a person might need to regulate the impulse to belch or scratch his backside during conversations with others or in talking to a group of people.

SOCIAL INTERACTION SKILLS RELATED TO SHAPING THE CONTENT OF SOCIAL INTERACTION

Questions

During conversation, the ability to question or to ask for information or relevant facts or information related to the topic being discussed is part of successful social interaction. Questioning skillfully requires requesting information that is relevant and will support the purpose of the interaction (AOTA, 2014). This is part of collaborative and interactive conversations—each participant asking questions relevant to the people involved or the topic. This is also important for activities in which the participant must request information from others in order to engage in or complete the activity.

Replies

During conversation, the ability to reply is demonstrated when participants keep the conversation flowing by replying back to each other appropriately (AOTA, 2014). The participants might be replying to a question or comments either with another statement or comment or by asking a question. At times, the reply might be a simple utterance, such as "hmmm." Regardless of the type of response, the reciprocal actions of replying or responding to each other is what keeps a conversation going.

Discloses

During a conversation or interaction, disclosing occurs when a participant in the interaction reveals her feelings, opinions, or private information about herself or others. This must be done in a manner that is socially appropriate for the situation and those involved in the interaction (AOTA, 2014). Activities that require a person to disclose things are those in which personal or private information must be shared. The timing of and manner in which disclosure occurs is dependent on the social demands and the context in which the interaction is occurring. In some social groups, if a person discloses very personal and deep emotions, it is welcomed and accepted. In other social groups, the same actions would not be so readily received.

Expresses Emotion

When a person expresses emotion during a conversation or interaction, he or she is demonstrating a variety of facial expressions and behaviors that convey emotion in a way that is socially appropriate (AOTA, 2014). The person's affect should reflect what is being discussed and be appropriate for the situation. For example, when discussing the death of a family member, it would be inappropriate for a participant in the discussion to grin widely or laugh. The expression of emotion is part of the interaction that occurs between participants in social engagement. The expression of emotion provides information to the participants as to the thoughts and feelings of others. We use the facial expressions of others to guide conversation. For example, in explaining a new concept to your friends, you would be able to discern, by their facial expressions, whether they understood or were completely perplexed. Activities that require the participants to express emotion are those in which the conversation or interactions rely on people's affect or demonstration of how they feel. This is also important in those social situations where a display of emotion is expected. For example, think of the expression of emotion that is socially expected at a funeral, a wedding, or upon receiving a gift.

Disagrees

During a conversation, there are times when participants may not agree with what is being said or discussed. To disagree, the person expresses his or her differences in opinion in a socially acceptable, appropriate manner (AOTA, 2014). What is acceptable and appropriate relies heavily on the social demands and the social context in which the interaction is occurring. In some situations, disagreeing with the person speaking might be very inappropriate. For example, if you were sitting in church or a synagogue and the priest or rabbi said something that you did not agree with, it would not be appropriate for you to stand up and speak out against what was being said. However, in a private conversation with a good friend, it might be very acceptable to disagree. This skill requires being able to determine when and how to disagree with what is being discussed. This skill is required in situations where there are social demands that limit how much or in what ways participants may express their differences in opinion.

Thanks

When we receive a gift, a compliment, or a services, offering thanks requires that we use socially appropriate words or gestures to acknowledge our appreciation (AOTA, 2014). This skill requires that the participant understand the social expectations of the context and respond appropriately to others. This is especially important for activities in which the participant will be receiving something, either a gift or services. The participant must be able to express gratitude not only verbally, but also through gestures and affect. For example, when you order food at a restaurant and the waiter or waitress brings your food, it is polite to say "thank you." Depending on the social context, the expectations of demonstrating thanks may extend beyond verbal expression and include physical expressions such as eye contact, a smile, or giving another person a hug.

SOCIAL INTERACTION SKILLS RELATED TO MAINTAINING THE FLOW OF SOCIAL INTERACTION

Transitions

During conversation, the topics can change or shift without the conversation ending. This requires the skill of being able to transition from one topic to another smoothly and without causing disruption in the conversation (AOTA, 2014). This is demonstrated by the speaker who guides the topics of conversation from one to another, as well as the listener who must be able to handle the change of topic. This dynamic shift from one topic to the next occurs often in casual conversations in a variety of social groups. The ability to transition from one topic to the other allows the participants to follow along and continue to be engaged in the interaction.

Times Response

During interactions with others, the exchange of information occurs in a reciprocal manner. In order for these replies or responses to occur at the appropriate time, without hesitation or interruptions, the speaker must time responses (AOTA, 2014). Speaking at the appropriate time is a social demand of many activities that involve reciprocal interactions. For example, when one is ordering food at a restaurant, the waiter or waitress might come to the table and explain the specials for the day. The customers time their responses so that they allow the waiter or waitress to finish before stating what they would like to order.

Times Duration

You may be able to think of a time where you asked a person a question and his or her answer took much longer that it should have, to the point where you wondered if this person were ever going to stop talking. Or maybe you have had the opposite experience; you asked a person a complex question and he or she gave you a simple one word answer, such as yes or no. The ability to speak for the appropriate and reasonable amount of time, based on the complexity of what needs to be expressed, is the ability to time duration

(AOTA, 2014). The extent to which the ability to time the duration of speech is dependent on the content of the information to be expressed and the social demands of the situations. In some situations, such as a job interview, it will be important that the interviewee be able to time the duration of his or her answers, so that the interviewer obtains enough information in a reasonable amount of time but not extraneous or irrelevant detail.

Takes Turns

When they are engaged in a reciprocal conversation, the participants take turns, giving each partner the freedom to speak or engage in the conversation (AOTA, 2014). This skill requires that each person take pauses so as to allow others to speak or interact. Taking turns requires allowing each person involved time to speak and not dominating the conversation. In social activities where more than one person is engaged in the conversation or where there is an expectation of reciprocal communication, the skill of taking turns will be required.

SOCIAL INTERACTION SKILLS RELATED TO VERBALLY SUPPORTING SOCIAL INTERACTION

Matches Language

It would not make sense to walk down the street and go into a grocery store and begin talking to the cashier using sign language. Nor would it make sense to yell or speak to that person in a very loud voice. Depending on the activity and the context of the activity, we match language, using a socially appropriate voice, tone, and dialect. Matching language also includes choosing a level of language that matches the abilities of our social partner (AOTA, 2014). This is especially important when the social demands of an activity specify the type of language to be used during social interactions. For example, in a church or synagogue, the language expected is of a low volume and involves the respectful use of words (no foul language). In a typical bar or club, on the other hand, the volume and pitch would be very different. Choosing a language level that meets the abilities and level of understanding of one's social partners is important, especially when communicating or interacting with others of a different age or cognitive level than your own. In communicating with a child, the pitch of speech and choice of words used are very different from those used in speaking with an adult.

Clarifies

During an interaction, there are times when one or more of the social partners does not understand or comprehend what is being communicated. It is at those times that a participant (or multiple participants) in the conversation may communicate nonverbally, use gestures, or express verbal messages signaling that they do not understand. A person clarifies when he or she responds to those cues and reacts, ensuring that the social partner or partners understand and can follow the conversation (AOTA, 2014). This occurs in reciprocal conversations or when new or difficulty information is being conveyed. This skill is highly required when any teaching or instruction occurs.

Acknowledges and Encourages

When engaged in reciprocal conversations, to acknowledge and encourage is a skill that requires the participants to acknowledge when something is expressed and encourage each participant to engage in the conversation. This also includes the skills of encouraging the conversation to continue or encouraging the social partner to continue to engage (AOTA, 2014). This skill is commonly expressed by nonverbal means such a nod or a shrug. Think of a conversation you have recently had. How did you know that he or she heard what you were saying? What verbal or nonverbal communication was used that encouraged you to continue to speak? We often use this skill without consciously thinking about it. Without it, however, we would have short-lived and unproductive conversations that would end prematurely.

Empathizes

To empasize during an interaction with others is to express a "supportive attitude toward the social partner by agreeing with, empathizing with, or expressing understanding of the social partner's feelings and experiences" (AOTA, 2014, p. S26). This skill is required when the topic of conversation is personal or controversial or is emotionally laden. In interactions where one social partner is expressing hurt feelings or personal difficulties, the others involved in the interaction should empathize by being supportive in their words and actions and conveying an understanding of the speaker's feelings. Empathizing can occur through verbal and nonverbal communication. A hand on a shoulder of someone who is crying is an example of how empathy can be shown nonverbally. A person's affect and how she positions her body also conveys empathy. Support and understanding can come from the choice of words as well, all of which should demonstrate a caring attitude.

SOCIAL INTERACTION SKILLS RELATED TO ADAPTING TO SOCIAL INTERACTION

Heeds

In order to achieve the goal of a conversation, the participants must heed to the intended purpose of the interaction. This means they must use goal-directed actions, speech, and behaviors that are focused on the intent of the interaction (AOTA, 2014). Basically, this means that the participants must stay on topic. During conversations, it is common for multiple topics to emerge. As the participants discuss these topics, they must pay heed to the current focus of discussion (i.e., they must stay focused on the topic at hand). This is especially important when a particular outcome is expected of the interaction. The ability to heed might be essential in working as a team on a project for school or work where an end product is expected from the interactions.

Accommodates

Earlier in this chapter, we discussed the process skill of accommodates, which was the skill of preventing inaccurate or ineffective task performance (AOTA, 2014). Much like the process skill of accommodates, the social interaction skill also involves preventing ineffective actions or behaviors. The social interaction skill of accommodates involves preventing socially inappropriate or ineffective social communication or interactions (AOTA, 2014). This means that the actions, words, or nonverbal expressions are modified as needed to prevent errors in communication, miscommunication, or social disruption. We might accommodate our reaction to someone who is revealing something shocking based on the social norms and expectations, so that we do not behave in a socially inappropriate way. For example, during a job interview, the interviewee must accommodate his or her language and behavior to the situation and the interviewer's behaviors and expectations.

Benefits

There is also a process skill called benefits, which was discussed earlier in this chapter. Much like the process skill, the social interaction skill of benefits involves preventing the recurrence of ineffective or inappropriate communication or interaction from occurring. To benefit means that a person learns from a previous mistake and prevents it from occurring again. In social interaction, one might behave a certain way and find that the behavior is not effective or socially acceptable (AOTA, 2014). One can benefit from such an incident by making sure that the ineffective behavior does not occur again (Activity 8-1).

ACTIVITY 8-1

List at least five activities that require a high level of social interaction skills. List the specific skills required.

_____

_____

_____

_____

_____

CONCLUSION

Performance skills are observable actions that people demonstrate while engaged in an activity or occupation. As OT practitioners, we evaluate and assess our clients' performance on a daily basis. We observe their performance, looking for ways in which they might improve. By understanding the level of skill required for an activity, we have a basis whereby to better understand how performance may be changed. Perhaps it is the environment or the occupation that influences performance. In this chapter, we looked at performance skills not from the perspective of evaluating a client's skill level, but rather by analyzing the degree of skill required for an activity. Being able to look at occupations and activities from both perspectives helps clinicians to understand how they might support greater participation.

QUESTIONS

1. How are performance skills different from body functions?
2. How do we determine how much skill is needed for an activity?
3. What external factors can influence the skill level required of our clients?
4. How do OT practitioners use performance skills in practice?
5. Name an activity that requires high levels of all performance skills.

ACTIVITIES

1. Continue to analyze the activity of washing hair in the shower by completing Activity 8-2.
2. Analyze the occupation you have been working on throughout this book, using section 11 of the Occupation-Based Activity Analysis Form in Appendix B.
3. Choose an activity in which you engage every day that requires all three performance skill areas. Using Appendix B, section 11, analyze the performance skills required and determine which are required the most.

ACTIVITY 8-2

Determine the performance skills required of washing hair in the shower as it typically is done. Briefly describe how each of the performance skills is used and then indicate the extent to which each is challenged. If a performance skill is not required at all during the activity, check off "none" and leave that row blank.

SKILL	NONE	LOW	MOD	HIGH	EXAMPLES OF HOW SKILL IS USED
Motor Skills					
Aligns					
Stabilizes					
Positions					
Reaches					
Bends					
Grips					
Manipulates					
Coordinates					
Moves					
Lifts					
Walks					
Transports					
Calibrates					
Flows					
Endures					
Paces					
Process Skills					
Paces					
Attends					
Heeds					
Chooses					
Uses					
Handles					
Inquires					
Initiates					
Continues					
Sequences					
Terminates					
Searches/locates					
Gathers					
Organizes					

(continued)

ACTIVITY 8-2 (CONTINUED)

SKILL	NONE	LOW	MOD	HIGH	EXAMPLES OF HOW SKILL IS USED
Process Skills					
Restores					
Navigates					
Notices/responds					
Adjusts					
Accommodates					
Benefits					
Social Interaction Skills					
Approaches/starts					
Concludes/disengages					
Produces speech					
Gesticulates					
Speaks fluently					
Turns toward					
Looks					
Places self					
Touches					
Regulates					
Questions					
Replies					
Discloses					
Expresses emotion					
Disagrees					
Thanks					
Transitions					
Times response					
Times duration					
Takes turns					
Matches language					
Clarifies					
Acknowledges and encourages					
Empathizes					
Heeds					
Accommodates					
Benefits					

REFERENCES

American Occupational Therapy Association. (2014). Occupational therapy practice framework. Domain and process (3rd ed.). *American Journal of Occupational Therapy, 68*(Suppl. 1), S1-S48. Retrieved from http.//dx.doi.org/10.5014/ajot.2014.682006

Boyt Schell, B., Gillen, G., & Scaffa, M. (2104). In B. A. Boyt Schell, G. Gillen, & M. Scaffa (Eds.), *Willard and Spackman's occupational therapy* (12th ed., pp. 1229-1243). Philadelphia, PA: Lippincott Williams & Wilkins.

Fisher, A. G., Bryze, K., Hume, V., & Griswold, L. A. (2007). *School AMPS. School version of the assessment of motor and process skills* (2nd ed.). Fort Collins, CO: Three Star Press.

Fisher, A. G., & Griswold, L. A. (2010). *Evaluation of social interaction* (2nd ed.). Fort Collins, CO: Three Star Press.

Fisher, A. G., & Jones, K. B. (2011a). *Assessment of motor and process skills. Development, standardization, and administration manual* (7th ed. rev.). Fort Collins, CO: Three Star Press.

Fisher, A. G., & Jones, K. B. (2011b). *Assessment of motor and process skills: User's manual* (7th ed. rev.). Fort Collins, CO: Three Star Press.

Mosby's dictionary of medicine, nursing & health professions (2006). St. Louis, MO: Author.

Simmons, C. D., Griswold, L. A., & Brett, B. (2010). Evaluation of social interaction during occupational engagement. *The American Journal of Occupational Therapy, 64*(1), 10-17.

Instructors: Have students watch the videos located with the supplemental materials at www.efacultylounge.com. After watching the videos, require students to complete sections 6, 8, and 9 of the activity analysis form in Appendix A.

Activity Analysis for Evaluation, Intervention Planning, and Outcomes

OBJECTIVES

- Identify the eight outcomes described in the *Framework* and how activity analysis is utilized as part of attaining those outcomes.
- Describe the approaches to intervention described in the *Framework* and how activity analysis plays a role in each.
- Define what grading of an activity means and how it is used in OT.
- Describe how to grade an activity up or down and when each is relevant.
- Understand the concept of scaffolding and how it is used in OT practice.
- Identify how to adapt activities and occupations in each of the activity demand areas.
- Understand how adapting and grading of activities are used to reach common outcomes in OT practice.

One of the unique contributions that OT brings to health care is the use of occupations as an intervention modality and the ability to adapt those occupations to allow for greater participation in daily life activities. Activity analysis is part of the process of evaluation and intervention (AOTA, 2014). Understanding the demands of the activities in which a client wants or needs to participate gives us insight into what our client needs to be able to do, as well as what the environmental considerations are.

During the OT evaluation process, the practitioner gains insight into the nature of the occupations that are meaningful to the client, as well as what defines successful completion of the occupation, the objects and properties required, the space demands, the client factors, and the performance skills required. This information is gleamed through an occupational profile and through objective observation and data gathering. It is through this process that goals and outcomes are established. Based on the intended outcomes, the clinician chooses appropriate approaches to intervention. This chapter provides a look at the different ways in which an activity analysis is utilized through both the evaluation and intervention process as detailed in the Outcomes and Approaches sections of the *Framework*.

Thomas H.
Occupation-Based Activity Analysis, Second Edition (pp 179-188).
© 2015 SLACK Incorporated.

OUTCOMES AND THE USE OF ACTIVITY ANALYSIS

Table 10 of the *Framework* (AOTA, 2014) defines eight broad outcomes of OT intervention: occupational performance, health and wellness, participation, prevention, quality of life, role competence, well-being, and occupational justice. The desired outcome for a client helps determine the approach the clinician should take. Outcomes are "the end result of the occupational therapy process" (AOTA, 2014, p. S34). We set outcomes during the evaluation process, setting treatment goals so that we can monitor the effects of intervention. The possible outcomes of occupational therapy describe what consumers of occupational therapy can potentially achieve. The list of outcomes provided in the *Framework* is broad but is not intended to be all-inclusive (AOTA, 2014).

Occupational Performance

Improved or enhanced occupational performance is one of the leading outcomes of OT practice. It is used when there is an inability to perform needed occupations or a limitation in being able to perform or if performance could be improved. If occupational performance is used as an outcome for a client, the result of the therapy provided leads to the ability to engage in, or the improved ability to engage in, occupations or activities. Improvement of occupational performance is an outcome that is set when there is a deficit or limitation in current performance. This applies to a broad spectrum of diagnoses and populations. A person who has had a stroke and lost the use of his or her right arm may work toward regaining the ability to dress and bathe himself. A woman with schizophrenia may work to improve her social interaction skills. Enhancement of occupational performance is used when the client is currently able to engage in his or her daily occupations, but performance could improve with targeted intervention.

An understanding of the demands of the activities that the practitioner and client are intending to improve or enhance allows the practitioner to establish intervention strategies focused on areas that can be improved or adapted. Grading and scaffolding of activities is very often utilized with this approach

to gradually improve a person's ability to complete activities on his or her own (this is discussed later in the chapter). Changes in occupational performance stem from improvements in performance skills, body functions, habits, and routines.

Health and Wellness

Health and wellness are outcomes that have been separately defined but aptly put together as an outcome measure. Health is defined as "a state of physical, mental, and social well-being, as well as a positive concept emphasizing social and person resources and physical capacities" (AOTA, 2014, p. S34). As an outcome, it means that OT practitioners help clients reach not only a state of physical well-being and optimal use of physical abilities, but also a positive mental and social state. Achieving wellness occurs when the client actively makes efforts toward a balanced and "successful existence" (AOTA, 2014, p. S34). This does not mean there is a lack of disease or disorder, but rather that the client attains a full and flourishing life. Health and wellness as an outcome is utilized with those who have a disability or illness, as well as those who do not. An example of this type of outcome would be a recently retired man taking lessons to learn to play the piano, something he had always wanted to do. The modification or adaptation of habits and routines can be part of the intervention process leading to this outcome. Activity analysis principles can be used in order to identify those activities that will lead to a greater sense of well-being for the client.

Participation

Simply put, participation as an outcome is the act of doing an occupation. Successful attainment of this type of outcome is achieved when clients engage in occupations that are meaningful and personally satisfying to them. Again, this outcome does not apply only to those with a disability or illness, but rather to all people actually engaging in meaningful occupations. An example of this would be to have a busy working father spend time playing baseball with his son. Practitioners can utilize activity analysis to determine barriers to participation, removing or adapting those activity demands that prevent successful participation.

Prevention

Prevention as an outcome focuses on thwarting those things that might impede a healthy life. As the opponent of illness and injury, health as a preventative measure stems from several factors at a personal, social, and environmental level. The *Framework* uses health education and promotion to reduce or prevent injury, illness, or the onset of unhealthy situations (AOTA, 2014). Preventing decline in any of these areas at a personal or societal level requires the OT practitioner to be able to analyze occupations and understand the complex interaction between the environment, human occupations, and performance. In order to promote a healthy lifestyle, the environment, objects, or actions required may need to be modified or adapted, changing aspects of how occupations are performed, the space or materials utilized, or the actions required. An example of this would be an educational support group for the caregivers of individuals with Alzheimer's disease to promote peace and physical well-being and prevent illness or familial unrest at home. This may include providing suggestions on how to adapt the home or tasks to decrease frustrations and safety hazards.

Quality of Life

Improved quality of life as an OT outcome involves understanding the client's perceived satisfaction with life, hope, self-concept, socioeconomic factors, and overall health and functioning (AOTA, 2014). Life satisfaction is a person's perception of "progress toward one's goals" (AOTA, 2014, p. S35). Having hope is the belief that reaching a goal is possible. Self-concept is what people believe to be true about themselves and their overall feelings about themselves. The first thing that people often associate with quality of life is health and functioning, which is not only physical health, but also the ability to complete self-care and to provide for oneself through work (AOTA, 2014). The achievement of this as an outcome can be demonstrated in a multitude of ways, from providing a workshop environment for cognitively impaired adolescents to begin teaching work skills at summer day camps for children with working parents. The activity analysis skills of a practitioner can be extremely helpful in addressing quality-of-life outcomes. Determining which activities or occupations have the characteristics that will lend toward improving a client's life will require the ability

to see the detailed therapeutic qualities of activities. For example, a practitioner might engage the client in creating a daily schedule that includes sensory experiences designed to provide the client with time throughout the day for relaxation (such as washing his or her hands in warm water). The clinician will determine these activities by analyzing the sensory properties of different activities in order to find those that provide the needed sensory experiences and fit within the client's contexts.

Role Competence

Roles are the behaviors expected by society or culture, based on the position the person has within familial or social contexts (AOTA, 2014). A woman may play many different roles in her daily life, such as mother, student, wife, church member, and daughter. Meeting role competence is the ability to "effectively meet the demands of roles in which the client engages" (AOTA, 2014, p. S35). An example of this would be if a mother with depression implemented bonding techniques with her baby (Figure 9-1). Role competence can be enabled by adapting aspects of the activity demands to allow for a greater ability to complete the activities needed to fulfill roles. For example, a worker may adapt his work station so that there are fewer distractions so as to improve his productivity (his role as an employee).

Well-Being

Well-being exists when a person is content with his or her own health, security, sense of belonging, and self-esteem. It also means that people who enjoy well-being are content with the opportunities they have for self-determination, roles, meaning in their lives, and the ability to help others (AOTA, 2014). Well-being is defined by the WHO (2006) as "a general term encompassing the total universe of human life domains, including physical, mental and social aspects" (p. 211). An example of this would be if a client with terminal cancer were able to find fulfillment in leaving a legacy for his sons by creating videos for their birthdays. The practitioner working with this client will analyze the activities the client needed to do, adapting the demands of the activities as necessary to allow for a greater sense of well-being on the part of the client.

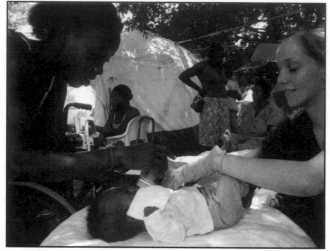

Figure 9-1. An OT student teaches infant-mother bonding techniques.

Occupational Justice

Occupational justice refers to having access to and being able to participate in occupations that are meaningful. Every person should have access to occupations that satisfy health, societal, and personal needs. For many, this means having access to resources or being allowed inclusion within social contexts (AOTA, 2014). For example, men and women in prisons have very little access to occupations that provide any personal meaning to them. An example of an occupational justice outcome would be the establishment of a free computer lab with adapted computer keyboards and mouse alternatives, enabling those with disabilities to use the Internet. Working to attain occupational justice for those who do not enjoy it requires creativity and determination on the part of OT practitioners. They must be able to look at all aspects of the activities or occupations their clients need or want to participate in and determine the barriers to engagement. By understanding what aspects of the activity demands are limited, the clinician can create strategies to overcome those limitations or create adaptations to reduce or eliminate the inequality to access.

APPROACHES TO INTERVENTION AND ACTIVITY ANALYSIS

How we help our clients meet their goals and planned outcomes relies on the approaches we used during intervention. The approaches used are based on multiple factors, such as the client's prognosis and impairment, the frames of reference or practice models being utilized by the practitioner, and the client's needs and preferences. The *Framework* delineates five different approaches to intervention. Each is unique and approaches the client's goals from a different perspective. Fundamental to the process of occupational therapy, activity analysis or occupation-based activity analysis is utilized with each of the approaches to intervention.

Create/Promote

This intervention approach is one that does not focus on or assume that there is a disability present in the client or the population receiving services. The focus of this approach is to provide "enriched contextual and activity experiences that will enhance performance" (AOTA, 2014, p. S33). Intervention using this approach utilizes natural contexts and activities that will improve engagement in occupations that are meaningful to the client. An example of this is providing parenting classes to couples who are adopting children from overseas to facilitate appropriate development through play and social activities. The interventions are not made in terms of a disability but rather to promote health. Using this approach, clients' occupations and activities are analyzed for areas that could be enhanced. Activities are also analyzed so that certain aspects of the activities can be adapted to allow for greater performance. The environment, objects, or social demands of specific activities can be modified to allow for enhanced engagement. For example, in creating activities for children being adopted from overseas, the clinician can think about activities that will promote bonding with the new parents. By critically analyzing and investigating different activities that challenge social interaction performance skills—such as looks, places self, touches—the clinician can provide activities that elicit and promote the use of these skills.

Establish/Restore

Intervention that utilizes the establish/restore approach is designed to change or restore client factors or skills or to help develop those skills that have not yet been established (AOTA, 2014). This approach uses activities and preparatory methods to help restore a skill after it has been lost because of a disability or injury. This approach also works to facilitate the development of skills or abilities that a client has not yet developed. For example, after a stroke, a clinician might use the establish/restore approach to help the client regain the use of a paralyzed or weakened upper extremity. A clinician working with a child who has a developmental disability might use the establish/restore approach to help the child develop social skills with his or her peers.

Central to the philosophy of OT is that the use of meaningful occupations can bring about change. Discerning what the therapeutic value of an activity or occupation is requires careful and detailed activity analysis. On the outside, our daily activities might appear to be mundane or even simple. After careful analysis, we can see that what might appear ordinary or mundane is actually quite complex. Take the activity of making scrambled eggs, which we have analyzed throughout the course of this book. After a thorough analysis, we find that this activity challenges the body functions of higher-level functions of cognition, attention, perception, sight, joint mobility, muscle power, and control of voluntary movement. It requires the motor skills of aligns, stabilizes, positions, reaches, grips, manipulates, coordinates, lifts, flows, and paces. It requires the process skills of paces, attends, heeds, chooses, uses, handles, continues, sequences, terminates, searches/locates, gathers, notices/responds, and adjusts. Thus we see that this activity promotes and challenges the further development of many body functions and performances skills.

OT practitioners utilizing the establish/restore approach rely on their skills of activity analysis to find therapeutic activities that will challenge and promote the use of client factors and performance skills needing further development or reestablishment. Finding the therapeutic value of an activity requires analyzing different activities, finding the client factors or performance skills that are most in demand, and using those activities during intervention to promote the client's further development. For example, if a client needs to develop his or her fine motor skills, the clinician using the establish/restore approach will find meaningful activities that call for the use of motor skills, thus providing a challenge to the client.

The "grading" of an activity up or down is a technique utilized in the establish/restore approach. Grading of an activity is used to increase or decrease the activity demands on the person while he or she is performing an activity. This is done incrementally to provide the "just-right challenge" and allow the person to develop the skills he or she needs while still

Figure 9-2. Grading can be compared to the grade of a hill.

ensuring his or her ultimate success. Grading down an activity is done by making the activity easier or providing assistance at difficult points so as to allow for success. Grading an activity down can be done by changing aspects of the activity demands, depending on where the client has difficulty. For example, if a child has difficulty with handwriting, we can grade down the activity by having him start with writing very large letters on paper with large lines. As he improves, we would grade up the activity by having him write smaller letters on smaller lines. To better understand the concepts of "grade up" and "grade down," think of the "steep grade" signs you see on the highway (Figure 9-2). If the grade is going down, the truck does not need to work as hard. Thus if you grade down an activity, the client does not have to struggle as much. If the grade is going uphill, the truck will struggle and work hard to get to the top of the hill. If you grade up an activity, you are making it more difficult (which you may do if you are looking to provide more of a challenge to your client).

Grading up an activity is often done in OT practice in order to provide a greater challenge to the client. For example, a client who is able to count out the correct change for an item may do well in the quiet environment of a therapy session, so the clinician can grade up the activity by having him or her do the activity while in a noisy grocery store. This is an appropriate way to grade up an activity as it matches the client's goals. Caution should be exercised in grading up an activity so that it does not cause undue frustration for the client, with little ties to desired outcomes. For example, if a client is working on being able to put books up on a bookshelf, a clinician could put weights around his or her wrists to make the activity more difficult.

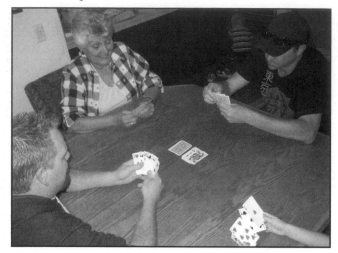

Figure 9-3. The activity of playing cards is one that may be graded up.

True, this is making the task more difficult, but the clinician should question the use of this and whether it is causing undue struggle and taking away from the point of the activity. Care should also be taken with not grading up too many aspects of the activity at one time. Providing the "just-right challenge" requires understanding what will provide a challenge to the client while still allowing him or her to be successful and not too frustrated. Think about how frustrated you would be if one of your teachers decided to grade up an assignment not by adding one addition piece to the assignment but by adding multiple parts. The same is true for your clients—they may become frustrated if too many new challenges are added all at one time.

Grading an activity begins with a good understanding of the activity's demands. What are the objects and properties being used? Can those be changed and made easier to use (or more difficult)? Can aspects of the environment be changed, such as the noise, temperature, working surface, or seating surface? How about the sequence and timing? Can the steps be changed or done in a different way? Perhaps the timing can be changed, allowing for more or less time to complete the activity. The social demands of an activity can be lessened by removing or changing the rules of the activity or decreasing the expectations of others. For example, Brent is having a hard time playing board games with others. His occupational therapist grades the activity down so that he can relearn how to participate in this occupation. She begins by having him play a simple game of solitaire, where there are no social demands on him. She grades up by having him play a card game with her. She further grades up by

adding another player to the game. As Brent improves, she adds social demands such as rules of behavior and interactions with the players (Figure 9-3).

To grade an activity, think first of which areas of the activity the client is struggling with. Is there a great amount of joint mobility of the hands required from a client who has limited range of motion? Having an understanding of how each of the activity demands will affect your client before he or she starts the activity will allow you to create ways to grade down the activity and allow your client to be successful. Once you have identified the required actions that the client is having difficulty with, you can choose to grade the activity down by providing scaffolding and changing the objects and properties, space demands, social demands, or sequence and timing. You can change the actions and skill level required by changing some of these activity demands or by providing assistance. Use Activity 9-1 to practice grading an activity.

Scaffolding is a method of grading an activity by providing assistance to the client when he or she might struggle or be unable to successfully complete a step. Think of when a child is beginning to learn how to feed him- or herself. The parent will hold his or her hand over the little hand that is holding the spoon. At first, the parent must guide the child's hand in scooping the food and bringing it to the child's mouth. Eventually, some of the support and assistance can be taken away when the child learns to bring the spoon to his or her mouth but continues to need help scooping the food. Little by little, the support (or scaffolding) is removed until the child is successful at completing the task without help (albeit with a bit of a mess). In this way, the activity begins as graded down but is slowly graded up as more challenge is given to the child and less to the parent. This technique is used frequently in OT sessions as a client learns or relearns an occupation. An example of this is when a person who has had a stroke must relearn how to put on a shirt, perhaps with the use of only one arm. As the person begins to learn how to do this activity, the clinician may need to provide a great amount of assistance in order for the client to get the shirt on. As the client learns how to do the activity, the clinician will provide fewer cues and less assistance so as to allow the client to become more independent. The clinician will need to think carefully about the amount of assistance given and be sure that with each trial, the scaffolding (or amount of support) is slowly taken away (Figure 9-4).

Activity 9-1

Describe how you would grade the activity of gardening by listing what you would change in each aspect of the activity demands.

ACTIVITY DEMAND	GRADE DOWN	GRADE UP
Objects and properties		
Space demands		
Social demands		
Sequence and timing		

Maintain

The maintain approach is one in which interventions are designed to preserve the client's abilities or body functions or their ability to meet their daily occupational needs. This approach is utilized when the client is at risk for a decrease in performance, health, or well-being (AOTA, 2014). An example of this is when OT practitioners provide home modification recommendations to older adults, which will then allow them to maintain their independence and remain in their homes as they age. Some intervention strategies using this approach are aimed at maintaining gains made during therapy. For example, a practitioner might instruct a client in range-of-motion exercises so that he or she can maintain the range of motion needed for everyday activities.

In order to maintain a specific aspect of a clients' performance, the OT practitioner must analyze the activities at risk of decline and find out which aspect of the activity demands can be supported by outside intervention. Sometimes the environment, space demands, or objects can be modified to allow for maintenance of performance, as in the example of the older adults attempting to remain independent at home. In the example of the client attempting to maintain range of motion of the shoulder, the practitioner would need to analyze and then recommend those activities or motions that would encourage shoulder motion.

Modify

The modify approach centers on changing or adapting the activity demands to allow for greater

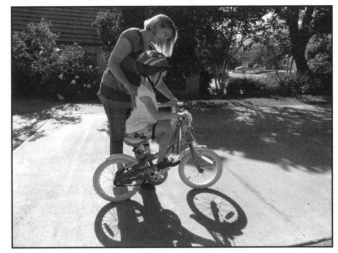

Figure 9-4. Using scaffolding, a mother helps her child learn how to ride a bike.

participation (AOTA, 2014). The demands of the activity can be changed by adapting the sequence and timing, objects or properties, space demands or environment, social demands, body functions, or performance skills required. How and why an occupation is changed in some way depends on the overall goal of intervention, the needs and desires of the client, and the theoretical approach the clinician is taking.

Adapting an activity is changing or modifying an aspect of the activity to allow for successful participation in an occupation (Crepeau & Schell, 2009). Adaptation requires thinking differently about an activity and finding an alternative way of getting it done. This requires flexibility on the part of the clinician and the client. While similar to grading in that we are changing aspects of the activity demands, in adapting an activity it is not with the intent to reduce or increase the demands on the client. The overall goal of adapting is to allow for greater participation and

---

ACTIVITY 9-2

Adapt the activity of making scrambled eggs by modifying aspects of the following activity demands.

ACTIVITY DEMAND	ADAPTATION/MODIFICATION
Objects and properties	
Space demands	
Social demands	
Sequence and timing	

---

independence. This could also include teaching compensatory techniques and having the client complete the activity differently (changing the sequence and timing). Modifying the amount of support and cues in the environment, such as providing visual cues or reminders, is also a way to adapt to allow for greater success.

An example of adapting is if a clinician provides a spoon with a built-up handle that allows someone with severe arthritis be feed him- or herself. If we go back to the example of the child struggling with handwriting, we can adapt certain aspects of the activity to allow him to be more successful immediately. We can change the height of the desk and chair he sits in (space demands) or give him a pencil with a bigger grip (objects and properties). The choice to adapt an activity is fed by many different factors, including the client's desired outcomes, openness to change, and diagnosis; time limitations; and the clinician's theoretical perspective. A clinician who has only one session with a client may choose to teach him or her how to adapt an activity to allow for greater independence immediately. The same is true of a client who has a progressive disease or one whose current body functions and structures will not improve. If the client's skill level is not likely to improve, the clinician may choose to adapt activities.

There are several areas of OT practice that have stemmed from the *modify* approach. Adaptive driving utilizes the concepts of adapting the objects and properties of the automobile, as well as providing drivers with adaptive methods that will allow them to be safe and independent. The entire field of assistive technology utilizes the modify approach to find adaptive methods and adaptive devices allowing access to telephones, computers, communication devices, and all other technological devices. In most fields of practice,

OT practitioners are seen as the experts in adapting, as we see the key to performance as not just within the client but as part of an interaction between the demands of the activity, the environment, and the client. Thus when aspects of the client cannot change or are slow to change, improved performance can be gained through adapting the activity or the environment.

To adapt or modify an activity, begin by listing the demands of the activity and listing the sequence and timing. Next, what body functions or performance skills are required for each step? Which of these are difficult for your client? Using this information, you can begin to determine those aspects of the activity that can be changed or adapted. Start with an aspect of the sequence or timing that could be changed. Could the client do things in a different order or with more time? Next, list the objects utilized. What could be modified—made bigger or smaller or changed in terms of its properties? What in the environment can be changed? Think not only about objects and access to things in the environment but also the sensory aspects; lighting and noise can make a huge difference in performance. Adapting and modifying activities can be very rewarding, as it challenges the practitioner to be creative and open-minded. As a result, a client may often become able to complete tasks that previously seemed difficult or impossible. Use Activity 9-2 to practice modifying an activity.

Prevent

OT intervention often focuses on preventing a decline in occupational performance. Using the prevent approach, practitioners focus on designing strategies that combat the formation or progression of injuries, illnesses, or occupational health difficulties.

This approach is utilized not only with people with disabilities, but also with those who are not disabled. The focus is on those who are at risk for problems in occupational performance (AOTA, 2014). For example, an OT practitioner might provide instruction in ergonomics and proper body mechanics to workers in a factory in order to prevent on-the-job injuries. OT services can be provided to expectant mothers who are on bed rest owing to an at-risk pregnancy, with the focus on preventing muscle atrophy, depression, and bed sores.

In order to design interventions to prevent decline or dysfunction, occupational therapists could utilize their activity analysis skills to determine which activities would be most likely to promote health or how to adapt the demands of the current activities to reduce risk. As discussed earlier, under the establish/restore approach, utilizing activities or occupations as agents of change requires understanding the therapeutic value of each activity, utilizing each activity with a thorough understanding of the unique challenges and benefits each provides. This is also true for the prevent approach. Using the example of the expectant mothers on bed rest, the OT practitioner will need to carefully choose activities that can provide challenges to the client, thus counteracting the risk of bed sores, depression, and muscle atrophy. Using the example of preventing injuries for workers in a factory, the OT practitioner might modify the work stations to be more ergonomically correct, recommend frequent stretch breaks, or recommend a modification in the way the workers lift and move. All of this requires an in-depth understanding of the demands of the activities the workers are required to complete. This includes thoroughly analyzing the environment and the objects being used. Prevention is a key part of OT practice, as it allows us to help our clients to remain healthy and injury free.

CONCLUSION

Activity analysis is a foundational and key aspect of the OT process, interwoven into evaluation and implantation of intervention. The outcomes outlined in the *Framework* provide a broad view of the potential end results of intervention. Activity analysis is one of the tools the OT practitioner can use to help meet client outcomes as set by the occupational therapist in the evaluation. The approaches we can take to address to reach the outcomes, create/promote, establish/restore, maintain, and modify/prevent all utilize aspects of activity analysis.

To meet client outcomes, adapting or grading of activities may be necessary. Changes can be made to make the activity easier and allow the client immediate performance or can be graded up slowly to allow for an increase in skill level. While grading of activities is primarily utilized when the desired outcome is occupational performance, it can be seen in all of the other types of outcomes as well. Through each of the types, adaptation can be found. Being able to see an activity from all aspects allows the clinician to find different ways in which it can be done. The modification of one aspect of an activity can address multiple outcomes. If a woman who uses a wheelchair has a baby that ends up in the neonatal intensive care unit, the occupational therapist can coach her to self-advocate for an adapted baby incubator, so that she will be able to reach inside and hold her baby. With the adaptation of the incubator, she has met health and wellness, participation, quality of life, role competence, well-being, and occupational justice outcomes.

ACTIVITIES

1. Design an intervention session for each of the outcomes described in the *Framework* and this chapter. What approaches would you use for each?

2. How would you adapt the activity of washing hair in the shower for limitations in the following body functions:
   a. Decreased joint mobility in the shoulder
   b. Decreased bilateral coordination
   c. Low vision
   d. Decreased fine motor control
   e. Decreased memory

3. Choose an occupation that is meaningful to you and teach it to your classmates. After the entire class has participated in the occupation, have each student list the body functions and performance skills this would help establish/restore, creating a list of therapeutic benefits.

4. Choose six different activities and set up a station for each, with all of the materials needed for each activity. Example of activities are playing a board game, washing windows, brushing teeth, making tea, and writing a letter to be sent in the mail. At

Activity 9-3

BODY FUNCTION REQUIRED	GRADE UP	GRADE DOWN
Ex: Joint mobility	Move handle bars forward so that greater forward reach is required	Build up the handles so that less range of motion in fingers is required
1.		
2.		
3.		
4.		
5.		

each station, place a piece of paper. On the left side of the paper, write "adaptation" and on the right, write "aspect." The students are to break up into groups and each to go to a station. They will be given 1 minute to brainstorm a way to adapt the activity. They will write it down on the sheet and then indicate what they are adapting: objects and properties used, the space, required actions, or social demands. They are to write down only one idea for adapting the activity. Once 1 minute has passed, the groups are to shift over to a different station and come up with a new idea for how to adapt the activity. Each group must read what has already been written down in order to not duplicate ideas. Once a group is unable to create a new idea, they are out of the game.

5. Make a list of ways in which to adapt the activity of washing hair in the shower. What aspects of the activity demands are you adapting?

Questions

1. What is the difference between the outcomes of enhancement of occupational performance and participation?
2. How are outcomes used in the OT process?
3. How are approaches used in the OT process?
4. What is the difference between grading and adapting?
5. At what times would it be appropriate to adapt an activity?

6. List the top five body functions challenged when riding a bike. List one way to grade up and one way to grade down for each of these body functions (Activity 9-3).
7. What are ways you might see scaffolding occurring with adults (not in a therapy setting)?

References

American Occupational Therapy Association. (2014). Occupational therapy practice framework: Domain and process (3rd ed.). *American Journal of Occupational Therapy, 68*(Suppl. 1), S1-S48. Retrieved from http://dx.doi.org/10.5014/ajot.2014.682006

Crepeau, E., & Schell, B. (2009). Analyzing occupations and activity. In E. Crepeau, E. Cohn, & B. Boyt Schell (Eds.), *Willard and Spackman's occupational therapy* (11th ed., pp. 359-374). Philadelphia, PA: Lippincott Williams & Wilkins.

Kroeneberg, F., Algado, S. S., & Pollard, N. (2005). *Occupational therapy without borders: Learning from the spirit of survivors.* Philadelphia, PA: Elsevier/Churchill Livingstone.

World Health Organization. (2006). Constitution of the World Health Organization (45th ed.). Retrieved from http://www.afro.who.int/index.php?option=com_docman&task=doc_download&dig=19&Itemid=2111WHO2006

3, Look at other analysises

2 precautions
2 contradictions

Appendix A

ACTIVITY ANALYSIS FORM

1. Occupation:

Area(s) of occupation for the client: Subcategory:

☐ Activities of daily living
☐ Instrumental activities of daily living
☐ Education
☐ Work
☐ Play
☐ Leisure
☐ Social participation

2. Objects and their properties required:

120 grit

wood stain (maple, oak)

3. Space demands:

4

4. Social demands:

5

(Chapter 5)

(Group focused)

(Individual focused)

Thomas H.
Occupation-Based Activity Analysis, Second Edition (pp 189-199).
© 2015 SLACK Incorporated.

→ elaborate / specific

5. Sequence and timing:

1. 10 minutes of sanding

2.

3.

4.

5.

6.

7.

8.

9.

10.

11.

12.

13.

14.

15.

[handwritten: Client factors Framework Chapter 6]

6. Body functions required:

[handwritten: ↗few checks if any → 1 example (words box)]

FUNCTION	NONE	MINIMALLY CHALLENGED	GREATLY CHALLENGED	HOW IT IS USED
Specific Mental Functions				
Higher-level cognitive: judgment, concept formation, metacognition, executive functions, praxis, cognitive flexibility, insight				
Attention: sustained attention and concentration; selective, divided, and shifting attention				
Memory: short-term, working, and long-term memory				
Perception: discrimination of sensations–auditory, tactile, visual, olfactory, gustatory, vestibular, and proprioceptive				
Thought: control and content of thought, awareness of reality, logical and coherent thought				
Sequencing complex movement: regulating speed, response, quality, and time of motor production				
Emotional: regulation and range of emotion, appropriateness of emotions				
Experience of self and time: appropriateness and range of emotion, body image, self-concept				
Global Mental Functions				
Consciousness: awareness and alertness, clarity and continuity of the wakeful state				
Orientation: orientation to person and self, place, time, and others				
Temperament and personality: extroversion, introversion, agreeableness, and conscientiousness; emotional stability; openness to experience; self-expression; confidence; motivation; self-control and impulse control; appetite				

FUNCTION	NONE	MINIMALLY CHALLENGED	GREATLY CHALLENGED	HOW IT IS USED
Global Mental Functions				
Energy and drive: motivation, impulse control, appetite				
Sleep: physiological process				
Sensory Functions				
Visual: quality of vision, visual acuity, visual stability, visual field				
Hearing: sound detection and discrimination, awareness of location and distance of sounds				
Vestibular: position, balance, secure movement against gravity				
Taste: qualities of bitterness, sweetness, sourness, and saltiness				
Smell: sensing odors and smells				
Proprioceptive: awareness of body position and space				
Touch: feeling of being touched, touching various textures				
Pain: localized and generalized pain				
Temperature and pressure: thermal awareness, sense of force applied to the skin				
Neuromusculoskeletal and Movement-Related Functions				
Joint mobility: joint range of motion				
Joint stability: structural integrity of joints				
Muscle Functions				
Muscle power: strength				
Muscle tone: degree of muscle tension				
Muscle endurance: sustaining muscle contraction				

FUNCTION	NONE	MINIMALLY CHALLENGED	GREATLY CHALLENGED	HOW IT IS USED
Movement Functions				
Motor reflexes: involuntary reflexes–involuntary contractions of muscles automatically induced by stretching				
Involuntary movement reactions: postural, body adjustment, and supporting reactions				
Control of voluntary movement: eye-hand and eye-foot coordination, bilateral integration, crossing midline, fine and gross motor control, oculomotor control				
Gait patterns: movements used to walk				
Cardiovascular, Hematological, Immunological, and Respiratory System Functions				
Cardiovascular system: blood pressure, heart rate and rhythm				
Hematological and immunological systems				
Respiratory system: rate, rhythm, and depth of respiration				
Additional functions of the cardiovascular and respiratory systems: physical endurance, stamina, aerobic capacity				
Voice and Speech; Digestive, Metabolic, and Endocrine Systems; and Genitourinary and Reproductive Systems Functions				
Voice and speech: rhythm and fluency, alternative vocalization functions				
Digestive, metabolic, and endocrine systems				
Genitourinary and reproductive systems: urinary, genital, and reproductive functions				
Skin and Related Structures Functions				
Skin: protection and repair				
Hair and nails				

7. Muscular analysis of movements required:

MUSCLE	NOT USED	MINIMALLY CHALLENGED	GREATLY CHALLENGED
Shoulder flexion			
Shoulder extension			
Shoulder abduction			
Shoulder adduction			
Shoulder internal rotation			
Shoulder external rotation			
Elbow flexion			
Elbow extension			
Wrist supination			
Wrist pronation			
Wrist flexion			
Wrist extension			
Thumb flexion			
Thumb abduction			
Finger flexion			
Finger extension			
Trunk flexion			
Trunk extension			
Trunk rotation			
Lower extremities			

8. Body structures required:

Chapter 7

CATEGORY	BODY STRUCTURE	REQUIRED? (CHECK IF YES)
Nervous system	Frontal lobe	
	Temporal lobe	
	Parietal lobe	
	Occipital lobe	
	Midbrain	
	Diencephalon	
	Basal ganglia	
	Cerebellum	
	Brainstem	
	Cranial nerves	
	Spinal cord	
	Spinal nerves	
	Meninges	
	Sympathetic nervous system	
	Parasympathetic nervous system	
Eyes, ears, and related structures	Eyeball: Conjunctiva, cornea, iris, retina, lens, vitreous body	
	Structures around eye: Lachrimal gland, eyelid, eyebrow, external ocular muscles	
	Structure of external ear	
	Structure of middle ear: Tympanic membrane, eustachian canal, ossicles	
	Structures of inner ear: Cochlea, vestibular labyrinth, semicircular canals, internal auditory meatus	
Voice and speech structures	Structures of the nose: External nose, nasal septum, nasal fossae	
	Structure of the mouth: Teeth, gums, hard palate, soft palate, tongue, lips	
	Structure of pharynx: Nasal pharynx and oral pharynx	
	Structure of larynx: Vocal folds	
Cardiovascular system	Heart: Atria, ventricles	
	Arteries	
	Veins	
	Capillaries	

CATEGORY	BODY STRUCTURE	REQUIRED? (CHECK IF YES)
Immunological system	Lymphatic vessels	
	Lymphatic nodes	
	Thymus	
	Spleen	
	Bone marrow	
Respiratory system	Trachea	
	Lungs: Bronchial tree, alveoli	
	Thoracic cage	
	Muscles of respiration: Intercostal muscles, diaphragm	
Digestive, metabolic, and endocrine systems	Salivary glands	
	Esophagus	
	Stomach	
	Intestines: Small and large	
	Pancreas	
	Liver	
	Gall bladder and ducts	
	Endocrine glands: Pituitary, thyroid, parathyroid, adrenal	
Genitourinary and reproductive systems	Urinary system: Kidneys, ureters, bladder, urethra	
	Structure of pelvic floor	
	Structure of reproductive system: Ovaries, uterus, breast and nipple, vagina and external genitalia, testes, penis, prostate	
Structures related to movement	Bones of cranium	
	Bones of face	
	Bones of neck region	
	Joints of head and neck	
	Bones of shoulder region	
	Joints of shoulder region	
	Muscles of shoulder region	
	Bones of upper arm	
	Elbow joint	
	Muscles of upper arm	
	Ligaments and fascia of upper arm	
	Bones of forearm	
	Wrist joint	
	Muscles of forearm	

CATEGORY	BODY STRUCTURE	REQUIRED? (CHECK IF YES)
Structures related to movement	Ligaments and fascia of forearm	
	Bones of hand	
	Joints of hand and fingers	
	Muscles of hand	
	Ligaments and fascia of hand	
	Bones of pelvic region	
	Joints of pelvic region	
	Muscles of pelvic region	
	Ligaments and fascia of pelvic region	
	Bones of thigh	
	Hip joint	
	Muscles of thigh	
	Ligaments and fascia of thigh	
	Bones of lower leg	
	Knee joint	
	Muscles of lower leg	
	Ligaments and fascia of lower leg	
	Bones of ankle and foot	
	Ankle, foot, and toe joints	
	Muscle of ankle and foot	
	Ligaments of fascia of ankle and foot	
	Cervical vertebral column	
	Lumbar vertebral column	
	Sacral vertebral column	
	Muscles of trunk	
	Ligaments and fascia of trunk	
Skin and related structures	Areas of skin: Head, neck, shoulder, upper extremity, pelvic region, lower extremities, trunk, and back	
	Structure of skin glands: Sweat and sebaceous	
	Structure of nails: Fingernails and toenails	
	Structure of hair	

Chapter 8

9. Performance skills required:

SKILL	NONE	LOW	MOD	HIGH	EXAMPLES OF HOW SKILL IS USED
Motor skills					
Aligns					
Stabilizes					
Positions					
Reaches					
Bends					
Grips					
Manipulates					
Coordinates					
Moves					
Lifts					
Walks					
Transports					
Calibrates					
Flows					
Endures					
Paces					
Process skills					
Paces					
Attends					
Heeds					
Chooses					
Uses					
Handles					
Inquires					
Initiates					
Continues					
Sequences					
Terminates					
Searches/locates					
Gathers					
Organizes					
Restores					

SKILL	NONE	LOW	MOD	HIGH	EXAMPLES OF HOW SKILL IS USED
Process skills					
Navigates					
Notices/responds					
Adjusts					
Accommodates					
Benefits					
Social interaction skills					
Approaches/ starts					
Concludes/disengages					
Produces speech					
Gesticulates					
Speaks fluently					
Turns toward					
Looks					
Places self					
Touches					
Regulates					
Questions					
Replies					
Discloses					
Expresses emotion					
Disagrees					
Thanks					
Transitions					
Times response					
Times duration					
Takes turns					
Matches language					
Clarifies					
Acknowledges and encourages					
Empathizes					
Heeds					
Accommodates					
Benefits					

Appendix B

OCCUPATION-BASED ACTIVITY ANALYSIS FORM

Complete the following occupation-based activity analysis on an occupation that is meaningful to you.

1. Occupation:

Area(s) of occupation for the client: Subcategory:

- ☐ Activities of daily living
- ☐ Instrumental activities of daily living
- ☐ Education
- ☐ Work
- ☐ Play
- ☐ Leisure
- ☐ Social participation

2. Values, beliefs, and spirituality associated with participation:

3. Contexts and environments: Indicate how each supports or inhibits participation in this occupation:

CONTEXT	SUPPORTS	INHIBITS
Cultural		
Personal		
Temporal		
Virtual		
Physical		
Social		

Thomas H.
Occupation-Based Activity Analysis, Second Edition (pp 201-211).
© 2015 SLACK Incorporated.

4. Performance patterns:

Parts of this occupation have elements of which of the following? (check all that apply):

PATTERN	DESCRIBE
Useful habit	
Dominating habit	
Routine	
Rituals	
Roles	

5. Objects and their properties required:

6. Social demands:

7. Sequence and timing:

1.

2.

3.

4.

5.

6.

7.

8.

9.

10.

11.

12.

13.

14.

15.

8. Muscular analysis:

MUSCLE	NOT USED	MINIMALLY CHALLENGED	GREATLY CHALLENGED
Shoulder flexion			
Shoulder extension			
Shoulder abduction			
Shoulder adduction			
Shoulder internal rotation			
Shoulder external rotation			
Elbow flexion			
Elbow extension			
Wrist supination			
Wrist pronation			
Wrist flexion			
Wrist extension			
Thumb flexion			
Thumb abduction			
Finger flexion			
Finger extension			
Trunk flexion			
Trunk extension			
Trunk rotation			
Lower extremities			

9. Identify body functions required:

FUNCTION	NONE	MINIMALLY CHALLENGED	GREATLY CHALLENGED	HOW IT IS USED
Specific Mental Functions				
Higher-level cognitive: judgment, concept formation, metacognition, executive functions, praxis, cognitive flexibility, insight				
Attention: sustained attention and concentration; selective, divided, and shifting attention				
Memory: short-term, working, and long-term memory				
Perception: discrimination of sensations–auditory, tactile, visual, olfactory, gustatory, vestibular, and proprioceptive				
Thought: control and content of thought, awareness of reality, logical and coherent thought				
Sequencing complex movement: regulating speed, response, quality, and time of motor production				
Emotional: regulation and range of emotion, appropriateness of emotions				
Experience of self and time: appropriateness and range of emotion, body image, self-concept				
Global Mental Functions				
Consciousness: awareness and alertness, clarity and continuity of the wakeful state				
Orientation: orientation to person and self, place, time, and others				
Temperament and personality: extroversion, introversion, agreeableness, and conscientiousness; emotional stability; openness to experience; self-expression; confidence; motivation; self-control and impulse control; appetite				

FUNCTION	NONE	MINIMALLY CHALLENGED	GREATLY CHALLENGED	HOW IT IS USED
Global Mental Functions				
Energy and drive: motivation, impulse control, appetite				
Sleep: physiological process				
Sensory Functions				
Visual: quality of vision, visual acuity, visual stability, visual field				
Hearing: sound detection and discrimination, awareness of location and distance of sounds				
Vestibular: position, balance, secure movement against gravity				
Taste: qualities of bitterness, sweetness, sourness, and saltiness				
Smell: sensing odors and smells				
Proprioceptive: awareness of body position and space				
Touch: feeling of being touched, touching various textures				
Pain: localized and generalized pain				
Temperature and pressure: thermal awareness, sense of force applied to skin				
Neuromusculoskeletal and Movement-Related Functions				
Joint mobility: joint range of motion				
Joint stability: structural integrity of joints				
Muscle Functions				
Muscle power: strength				
Muscle tone: degree of muscle tension				
Muscle endurance: sustaining muscle contraction				

FUNCTION	NONE	MINIMALLY CHALLENGED	GREATLY CHALLENGED	HOW IT IS USED
Movement Functions				
Motor reflexes: involuntary reflexes–involuntary contractions of muscles automatically induced by stretching				
Involuntary movement reactions: postural, body adjustment, and supporting reactions				
Control of voluntary movement: eye-hand and eye-foot coordination, bilateral integration, crossing midline, fine and gross motor control, oculomotor control				
Gait patterns: movements used to walk				
Cardiovascular, Hematological, Immunological, and Respiratory System Functions				
Cardiovascular system: blood pressure, heart rate and rhythm				
Hematological and immunological systems				
Respiratory system: rate, rhythm, depth of respiration				
Additional functions of the cardiovascular and respiratory systems: physical endurance, stamina, aerobic capacity				
Voice and Speech; Digestive, Metabolic, and Endocrine Systems; and Genitourinary and Reproductive Systems Functions				
Voice and speech: rhythm and fluency, alternative vocalization functions				
Digestive, metabolic, and endocrine systems				
Genitourinary and reproductive systems: urinary, genital, and reproductive functions				
Skin and Related Structures Functions				
Skin: protection and repair				
Hair and nails				

10. Body structures required:

CATEGORY	BODY STRUCTURE	REQUIRED? (CHECK IF YES)
Nervous system	Frontal lobe	
	Temporal lobe	
	Parietal lobe	
	Occipital lobe	
	Midbrain	
	Diencephalon	
	Basal ganglia	
	Cerebellum	
	Brainstem	
	Cranial nerves	
	Spinal cord	
	Spinal nerves	
	Meninges	
	Sympathetic nervous system	
	Parasympathetic nervous system	
Eyes, ears, and related structures	Eyeball: Conjunctiva, cornea, iris, retina, lens, vitreous body	
	Structures around eye: Lachrimal gland, eyelid, eyebrow, external ocular muscles	
	Structure of external ear	
	Structure of middle ear: Tympanic membrane, eustachian canal, ossicles	
	Structures of inner ear: Cochlea, vestibular labyrinth, semicircular canals, internal auditory meatus	
Voice and speech structures	Structures of the nose: External nose, nasal septum, nasal fossae	
	Structure of the mouth: Teeth, gums, hard palate, soft palate, tongue, lips	
	Structure of pharynx: Nasal pharynx and oral pharynx	
	Structure of larynx: Vocal folds	
Cardiovascular system	Heart: Atria, ventricles	
	Arteries	
	Veins	
	Capillaries	

CATEGORY	BODY STRUCTURE	REQUIRED? (CHECK IF YES)
Immunological system	Lymphatic vessels	
	Lymphatic nodes	
	Thymus	
	Spleen	
	Bone marrow	
Respiratory system	Trachea	
	Lungs: Bronchial tree, alveoli	
	Thoracic cage	
	Muscles of respiration: Intercostal muscles, diaphragm	
Digestive, metabolic, and endocrine systems	Salivary glands	
	Esophagus	
	Stomach	
	Intestines: Small and large	
	Pancreas	
	Liver	
	Gall bladder and ducts	
	Endocrine glands: Pituitary, thyroid, parathyroid, adrenal	
Genitourinary and reproductive systems	Urinary system: Kidneys, ureters, bladder, urethra	
	Structure of pelvic floor	
	Structure of reproductive system: Ovaries, uterus, breast and nipple, vagina and external genitalia, testes, penis, prostate	
Structures related to movement	Bones of cranium	
	Bones of face	
	Bones of neck region	
	Joints of head and neck	
	Bones of shoulder region	
	Joints of shoulder region	
	Muscles of shoulder region	
	Bones of upper arm	
	Elbow joint	
	Muscles of upper arm	
	Ligaments and fascia of upper arm	
	Bones of forearm	
	Wrist joint	
	Muscles of forearm	

CATEGORY	BODY STRUCTURE	REQUIRED? (CHECK IF YES)
Structures related to movement	Ligaments and fascia of forearm	
	Bones of hand	
	Joints of hand and fingers	
	Muscles of hand	
	Ligaments and fascia of hand	
	Bones of pelvic region	
	Joints of pelvic region	
	Muscles of pelvic region	
	Ligaments and fascia of pelvic region	
	Bones of thigh	
	Hip joint	
	Muscles of thigh	
	Ligaments and fascia of thigh	
	Bones of lower leg	
	Knee joint	
	Muscles of lower leg	
	Ligaments and fascia of lower leg	
	Bones of ankle and foot	
	Ankle, foot, and toe joints	
	Muscle of ankle and foot	
	Ligaments of fascia of ankle and foot	
	Cervical vertebral column	
	Lumbar vertebral column	
	Sacral vertebral column	
	Muscles of trunk	
	Ligaments and fascia of trunk	
Skin and related structures	Areas of skin: Head, neck, shoulder, upper extremity, pelvic region, lower extremities, trunk, and back	
	Structure of skin glands: Sweat and sebaceous	
	Structure of nails: Fingernails and toenails	
	Structure of hair	

11. Identify the performance skills required:

SKILL	NONE	LOW	MOD	HIGH	EXAMPLES OF HOW SKILL IS USED
Motor skills					
Aligns					
Stabilizes					
Positions					
Reaches					
Bends					
Grips					
Manipulates					
Coordinates					
Moves					
Lifts					
Walks					
Transports					
Calibrates					
Flows					
Endures					
Paces					
Process skills					
Paces					
Attends					
Heeds					
Chooses					
Uses					
Handles					
Inquires					
Initiates					
Continues					
Sequences					
Terminates					
Searches/locates					
Gathers					
Organizes					
Restores					

SKILL	NONE	LOW	MOD	HIGH	EXAMPLES OF HOW SKILL IS USED
Process skills					
Navigates					
Notices/responds					
Adjusts					
Accommodates					
Benefits					
Social interaction skills					
Approaches/ starts					
Concludes/disengages					
Produces speech					
Gesticulates					
Speaks fluently					
Turns toward					
Looks					
Places self					
Touches					
Regulates					
Questions					
Replies					
Discloses					
Expresses emotion					
Disagrees					
Thanks					
Transitions					
Times response					
Times duration					
Takes turns					
Matches language					
Clarifies					
Acknowledges and encourages					
Empathizes					
Heeds					
Accommodates					
Benefits					

Appendix C

COMPLETED ACTIVITY ANALYSIS FORM

1. Occupation:
Area(s) of occupation for the client:　　　　Subcategory:
　☐ Activities of daily living　　　　　　_____
　☐ Instrumental activities of daily living　Meal preparation_____
　☐ Education　　　　　　　　　　　　　_____
　☐ Work　　　　　　　　　　　　　　　_____
　☐ Play　　　　　　　　　　　　　　　_____
　☐ Leisure　　　　　　　　　　　　　　_____
　☐ Social participation　　　　　　　　　_____

2. Objects and their properties required:
　• Tools: Nonstick frying pan, plastic spatula, bowl, fork, plate
　• Materials: Two fresh eggs, nonstick spray
　• Equipment: Trash can, stove
　• (Properties are listed with each item)

3. Space demands:
　• Adequate lighting to see the eggs in the pan
　• Space to stand and move in front of the stove
　• Flat counter on which to set eggs, bowl, and spatula

4. Social demands:
　• Clean up after cooking
　• Eggs must be edible—not burned or undercooked
　• Must have permission to use the stove or kitchen
　• Wash hands before cooking
　• Do not stick hands into the eggs

Thomas H.
Occupation-Based Activity Analysis, Second Edition (pp 213-223).
© 2015 SLACK Incorporated.

5. Sequence and timing:
   1. Pick up the pan by grasping the handle of the pan with one hand and picking it up.
   2. Grasp the can of nonstick spray with the other hand.
   3. Hold the nozzle of the can over 6 inches above the pan.
   4. Press the nozzle down and spray the entire surface of the pan quickly.
   5. Set down the can of spray gently on the countertop.
   6. Place the pan on top of the burner.
   7. Turn on the burner of the stove by turning the burner knob to the right slowly until a clicking is heard.
   8. Turn the knob to the left slowly until the flame is at a medium level.
   9. Grasp one egg with one hand.
   10. Tap the egg against the edge of the counter until a crack is formed.
   11. Bring the egg above the pan quickly.
   12. Using both hands, place the thumbs into the crack and pull the shell apart gently, allowing the egg to fall into the bowl.
   13. Place the egg shell into the trashcan.
   14. Repeat steps 9 to 13 for the second egg.
   15. Hold the edge of the bowl gently with the left hand.
   16. Pick up the fork along the flat edge using the right hand.
   17. Place the fork into the bowl and move the fork in a circular motion quickly.
   18. Set the fork down onto the counter.
   19. Pour the eggs into the pan carefully.
   20. Grasp the handle of the pan with the left hand and pick up the spatula with the right hand.
   21. Holding the handle of the pan, stir the eggs slowly with the tip of the spatula.
   22. Continue to stir until the eggs are fluffy and no longer watery.
   23. Turn the knob of the stove to the off position until the flame goes out.
   24. Pick up the pan by grasping the handle of the pan and lifting it up carefully.
   25. Pick up the spatula by the handle.
   26. Tilt the pan over the plate and scrape the eggs out of the pan using the spatula.
   27. Set down the pan on the burner.
   28. Set down the spatula on the countertop.

6. Body functions required:

FUNCTION	NONE	MINIMALLY CHALLENGED	GREATLY CHALLENGED	HOW IT IS USED
Specific Mental Functions				
Higher-level cognitive: judgment, concept formation, metacognition, executive functions, praxis, cognitive flexibility, insight			X	Decide when to put eggs on pan, when eggs are done, when to use different burner if one doesn't start
Attention: sustained attention and concentration; selective, divided, and shifting attention			X	Keep attention on cooking eggs or they will burn
Memory: short-term, working, and long-term memory		X		Recall what steps have been completed; remember how to make scrambled eggs
Perception: discrimination of sensations–auditory, tactile, visual, olfactory, gustatory, vestibular, and proprioceptive			X	Feel with fingers the cracks in eggs to crack open; see where to put eggs; feel and see consistency
Thought: control and content of thought, awareness of reality, logical and coherent thought	X			
Sequencing complex movement: regulating speed, response, quality, and time of motor production		X		Stir or whisk eggs at appropriate speed; crack eggs and move into bowl
Emotional: regulation and range of emotion, appropriateness of emotions	X			
Experience of self and time: appropriateness of and range of emotion, body image, self-concept	X			
Global Mental Functions				
Consciousness: awareness and alertness, clarity and continuity of the wakeful state		X		Stay alert to environment and eggs during cooking
Orientation: orientation to person and self, place, time, and others		X		Know one is in a kitchen
Temperament and personality: extroversion, introversion, agreeableness, and conscientiousness; emotional stability; openness to experience; self-expression; confidence; motivation; self-control and impulse control; appetite	X			

FUNCTION	NONE	MINIMALLY CHALLENGED	GREATLY CHALLENGED	HOW IT IS USED
Global Mental Functions				
Energy and drive: motivation, impulse control, and appetite		X		Be motivated to complete cooking the eggs
Sleep: physiological process	X			
Sensory Functions				
Visual: quality of vision, visual acuity, visual stability, visual field			X	See all objects and equipment being used
Hearing: sound detection and discrimination, awareness of location and distance of sounds	X			
Vestibular: position, balance, secure movement against gravity		X		Stabilize body when moving from one position to next and lifting eggs
Taste: qualities of bitterness, sweetness, sourness, and saltiness	X			Only cooking eggs, not eating
Smell: sensing odors and smells		X		Smell when burning
Proprioceptive: awareness of body position and space		X		Move arms and trunk to pick up spatula, eggs, pan, plate; be aware of where body is and where it is moving
Touch: feeling of being touched, touching various textures		X		Feel crack in egg in order to break it open
Pain: localized and generalized pain	X			
Temperature and pressure: thermal awareness, sense of force applied to the skin		X		Sense when too close to pan or flame
Neuromusculoskeletal and Movement-Related Functions				
Joint mobility: joint range of motion		X		Grasp handle of pan and hold eggs
Joint stability: structural integrity of joints	X			
Muscle Functions				
Muscle power: strength		X		Stir eggs and strike them against surface; break eggs using fingers
Muscle tone: degree of muscle tension		X		Produce smooth movements when grasping and breaking eggs over bowl
Muscle endurance: sustaining muscle contraction		X		Sustain standing and stirring with one hand for several minutes

FUNCTION	NONE	MINIMALLY CHALLENGED	GREATLY CHALLENGED	HOW IT IS USED
Movement Functions				
Motor reflexes: involuntary reflexes–contractions of muscles automatically induced by stretching	X			
Involuntary movement reactions: postural, body adjustment, and supporting reactions	X			
Control of voluntary movement: eye-hand and eye-foot coordination, bilateral integration, crossing midline, fine and gross motor control, oculomotor control			X	Reach for spatula and eggs; crack eggs; stir; hold handle of pan while stirring eggs; pick up bowl or pan
Gait patterns: movements used to walk	X			
Cardiovascular, Hematological, Immunological, and Respiratory Systems Functions				
Cardiovascular systems: blood pressure, heart rate and rhythm	X			
Hematological and immunological systems	X			
Respiratory system: rate, rhythm, and depth of respiration	X			
Addition functions of the cardiovascular and respiratory systems: physical endurance, stamina, aerobic capacity		X		Stand and move for several minutes
Voice and Speech; Digestive, Metabolic, and Endocrine Systems; and Genitourinary and Reproductive Systems Functions				
Voice and speech: fluency and rhythm, alternative vocalization functions	X			
Digestive, metabolic, and endocrine systems	X			Not eating eggs, only cooking
Genitourinary and reproductive systems: urinary, genital, and reproductive functions	X			
Skin and Related Structures Functions				
Skin: protection and repair		X		Protect against sharp eggshell edges
Hair and nails	X			

7. Muscular analysis of movements required:

MUSCLE	NOT USED	MINIMALLY CHALLENGED	GREATLY CHALLENGED
Shoulder flexion		X	
Shoulder extension		X	
Shoulder abduction		X	
Shoulder adduction		X	
Shoulder internal rotation		X	
Shoulder external rotation		X	
Elbow flexion		X	
Elbow extension		X	
Wrist supination		X	
Wrist pronation		X	
Wrist flexion		X	
Wrist extension		X	
Thumb flexion		X	
Thumb abduction	X		
Finger flexion		X	
Finger extension		X	
Trunk flexion	X		
Trunk extension	X		
Trunk rotation		X	
Lower extremities		X	

8. Body structures required:

CATEGORY	BODY STRUCTURE	REQUIRED? (CHECK IF YES)
Nervous system	Frontal lobe	
	Temporal lobe	
	Parietal lobe	
	Occipital lobe	
	Midbrain	
	Diencephalon	
	Basal ganglia	
	Cerebellum	
	Brainstem	
	Cranial nerves	
	Spinal cord	
	Spinal nerves	
	Meninges	
	Sympathetic nervous system	
	Parasympathetic nervous system	
Eyes, ears, and related structures	Eyeball: Conjunctiva, cornea, iris, retina, lens, vitreous body	
	Structures around eye: Lachrimal gland, eyelid, eyebrow, external ocular muscles	
	Structure of external ear	
	Structure of middle ear: Tympanic membrane, eustachian canal, ossicles	
	Structures of inner ear: Cochlea, vestibular labyrinth, semicircular canals, internal auditory meatus	
Voice and speech structures	Structures of the nose: External nose, nasal septum, nasal fossae	
	Structure of the mouth: Teeth, gums, hard palate, soft palate, tongue, lips	
	Structure of pharynx: Nasal pharynx and oral pharynx	
	Structure of larynx: Vocal folds	
Cardiovascular system	Heart: Atria, ventricles	
	Arteries	
	Veins	
	Capillaries	

CATEGORY	BODY STRUCTURE	REQUIRED? (CHECK IF YES)
Immune system	Lymphatic vessels	
	Lymphatic nodes	
	Thymus	
	Spleen	
	Bone marrow	
Respiratory system	Trachea	
	Lungs: Bronchial tree, alveoli	
	Thoracic cage	
	Muscles of respiration: Intercostal muscles, diaphragm	
Digestive, metabolic, and endocrine systems	Salivary glands	
	Esophagus	
	Stomach	
	Intestines: Small and large	
	Pancreas	
	Liver	
	Gall bladder and ducts	
	Endocrine glands: Pituitary, thyroid, parathyroid, adrenal	
Genitourinary and repro- ductive systems	Urinary system: Kidneys, ureters, bladder, urethra	
	Structure of pelvic floor	
	Structure of reproductive system: Ovaries, uterus, breast and nip- ple, vagina and external genitalia, testes, penis, prostate	
Structures related to movement	Bones of cranium	
	Bones of face	
	Bones of neck region	
	Joints of head and neck	
	Bones of shoulder region	
	Joints of shoulder region	
	Muscles of shoulder region	
	Bones of upper arm	
	Elbow joint	
	Muscles of upper arm	
	Ligaments and fascia of upper arm	
	Bones of forearm	
	Wrist joint	
	Muscles of forearm	

CATEGORY	BODY STRUCTURE	REQUIRED? (CHECK IF YES)
Structures related to movement	Ligaments and fascia of forearm	
	Bones of hand	
	Joints of hand and fingers	
	Muscles of hand	
	Ligaments and fascia of hand	
	Bones of pelvic region	
	Joints of pelvic region	
	Muscles of pelvic region	
	Ligaments and fascia of pelvic region	
	Bones of thigh	
	Hip joint	
	Muscles of thigh	
	Ligaments and fascia of thigh	
	Bones of lower leg	
	Knee joint	
	Muscles of lower leg	
	Ligaments and fascia of lower leg	
	Bones of ankle and foot	
	Ankle, foot, and toe joints	
	Muscle of ankle and foot	
	Ligaments of fascia of ankle and foot	
	Cervical vertebral column	
	Lumbar vertebral column	
	Sacral vertebral column	
	Muscles of trunk	
	Ligaments and fascia of trunk	
Skin and related structures	Areas of skin: Head, neck, shoulder, upper extremity, pelvic region, lower extremities, trunk, and back	
	Structure of skin glands: Sweat and sebaceous	
	Structure of nails: Fingernails and toenails	
	Structure of hair	

9. Performance skills required:

SKILL	NONE	LOW	MOD	HIGH	EXAMPLES OF HOW SKILL IS USED
Motor skills					
Aligns			X		Stand at stove; use pan, spatula, eggs; hold body upright
Stabilizes			X		Move from one position at stove to another area; using spatula, pan, eggs
Positions			X		Place body in front of pan while cooking to effectively stir
Reaches			X		Pick up pan, eggs, spatula, bowl
Bends	X				
Grips			X		Hold the spatula when stirring, eggs when cracking, bowl when whisking
Manipulates			X		Turn on stove using buttons; manipulate eggs in hands to crack open
Coordinates			X		Use both hands to crack open eggs; hold handle of pan with one hand while stirring with the other
Moves		X			Move bowl toward pan
Lifts			X		Pick up eggs, spatula, pan, bowl
Walks		X			Move from stove to other area of kitchen
Transports		X			Carry eggs, bowl, spatula over to stove
Calibrates			X		Calibrate how hard to hit eggs on counter to break open and how fast to whisk or stir eggs
Flows		X			Stir eggs, put eggs into pan
Endures		X			Continue to stir eggs until cooked thoroughly
Paces	X				
Process skills					
Paces	X				
Attends			X		Assure eggs do not burn while cooking
Heeds			X		Continue until eggs are thoroughly cooked and out of pan
Chooses				X	Select correct utensils to cook eggs and complete task
Uses			X		Use spatula, whisk, pan, eggs as needed
Handles				X	Handle eggs with care without breaking them
Inquires	X				
Initiates			X		Continuously crack eggs, whisk, move to pan
Continues					Whisk until eggs are done; stir eggs until cooked thoroughly
Sequences					Put eggs into pan after it is preheated and eggs are mixed
Terminates				X	Stop whisking eggs when thoroughly mixed; stop cooking eggs when thoroughly cooked
Searches/locates			X		Find spatula, pan, bowl, eggs
Gathers			X		Place bowl and eggs near stove and spatula and pan at stove
Organizes		X			Place spatula and bowl in logical place next to pan on stove
Restores	X				

SKILL	NONE	LOW	MOD	HIGH	EXAMPLES OF HOW SKILL IS USED
Process skills					
Navigates		X			Move from stove to other areas of kitchen without bumping into things
Notices/responds			X		Respond to visual information about state of eggs cooking in pan and to feeling of heat
Adjusts		X			Turn heat up or down on stove based on how quickly or slowly eggs are cooking
Accommodates		X			Move handle of pan inward so it is not caught and causes pan to fall to floor; crack eggs over bowl so contents do not spill
Benefits	X				
Social interaction skills					
Approaches/starts	X				
Concludes/disengages	X				
Produces speech	X				
Gesticulates	X				
Speaks fluently	X				
Turns toward	X				
Looks	X				
Places self	X				
Touches	X				
Regulates	X				
Questions	X				
Replies	X				
Discloses	X				
Expresses emotion	X				
Disagrees	X				
Thanks	X				
Transitions	X				
Times response	X				
Times duration	X				
Takes turns	X				
Matches language	X				
Clarifies	X				
Acknowledges and encourages	X				
Empathizes	X				
Heeds	X				
Accommodates	X				
Benefits	X				

Index